VIRTUAL
MEDICINE

A new dimension in energy healing

Dr Keith Scott-Mumby

These new concepts of life and energy bring back a medicine
of humility before the miracle we call life. The art of
medicine becomes a practice composed of the life energies of
the physician, the patient and the Earth.

Dr Robert O. Becker, *Cross Currents: The Perils of
Electropollution, The Promise of Electromedicine*

Thorsons
An Imprint of HarperCollins*Publishers*

To Telly, who saw the dark hour when it was conceived,
and was there in the happy hour it was born.

Thorsons
An Imprint of HarperCollins*Publishers*
77–85 Fulham Palace Road,
Hammersmith, London W6 8JB

Published by Thorsons 1999
The Thorsons Website address is: www.thorsons.com

10 9 8 7 6 5 4 3 2 1

A catalogue record for this book
is available from the British Library

ISBN 0 7225 3823 5

Printed in Great Britain by
Creative Print and Design (Wales), Ebbw Vale

Contents

PREFACE

I hope this book will fascinate and delight the reader with new insights into age-old questions of disease, vitality and even death. It would fail if it did not at least shock some. You will see, in the chapters to come, that certain practitioners are able to detect life events beyond the confines of the body. That is to say that real-time phenomena, which once would have appeared magical, occult or 'etheric', can be identified using ordinary scientific equipment tuned to do so, devices which I have labelled as belonging to the domain of Virtual Medicine (or cyber-healing). If nothing else, this shows us that life is not merely a property of physical matter.

You will also learn that disease as we now know it is nothing more than the *final* result of events which have been going on in and around the body for a long period before anything is noticeably wrong. Once again, we can now witness these danger events in real-time, using advanced equipment to visualize them, and this opens up the possibility of successful 'treatment' before ever the disease becomes manifest. Here is another reason for using the term Virtual Medicine. It is healing at a higher and more intelligent dimension.

There is some discussion about what was called, earlier this century, the new physics – meaning the startling revelations of quantum mechanics and Einstein's mind-bending principles of Relativity. Add to that the powerful assertion of chaos as a governing principle of the dynamics we actually experience. Gradually science has had to adopt a new view of reality that was not much to its liking.

Einstein's famous equation, $e = mc^2$, has caused us to modify our view of particles and matter in an essential way. We had to start thinking of matter or 'stuff' as a property of energy. This means that matter can no longer be viewed as something static or permanent. It is equivalent to a certain amount of energy or process, which expresses itself in the form of something apparently tangible.

Then in almost contemporaneous development quantum

mechanics came along, with its strange sub-atomic world of probability fields and 'virtual particles' from the great quantum field. Particles just leapt into existence in this void and vanished again just as adroitly. Physics was beginning to sound more like witchcraft than science.

Then suddenly in the last quarter-century of this millennium we have discovered that our 'advanced physics' is beginning to meet ancient systems of the mind, such as *Tao* and the *Vedas*. That is to say, science is catching up with older wisdom, not the other way round. There is a remarkable and quite stirring concordance between texts written thousands of years ago and what scientists working at the leading edge of knowledge are discovering about today's reality. In the 1970s we saw books like *The Tao of Physics* by Fritjof Capra and *The Dancing Wu-Li Masters* by Gary Zukov which opened our eyes to the way particle physics was uncovering what appeared to be a conscious and intelligent universe, of which we were a part and therefore involved in all the rules.

As Fritjof Capra tells us in *The Tao of Physics*:

> The Eastern mystics see the universe as an inseparable web, whose interconnections are dynamic and not static. The cosmic web is alive; it moves grows and changes continually. Modern physics, too, has come to conceive of the universe as such a web of relations and, like Eastern mysticism, has recognized that the web is intrinsically dynamic.[11]

Despite this swing of emphasis and broadening of philosophy in the leading natural science of physics, medicine has consistently refused to tune in to the important new issues. If only doctors knew more physics they probably would not rant and rail against healing alternative disciplines quite as much as they do like to. Chemistry, biology and other disciplines all necessarily take their cues from physics, but not medicine, seemingly. Instead those doctors who wished to establish better healing values in this new domain were attacked, quite savagely at times, and denounced vituperatively as charlatans and snake-oil peddlers.

Well, I'm pleased to say that things have begun to change. We are seeing a rebirth of the philosophy of Vitalism, the understanding that the world we experience is structured and takes its cues from life itself and not from some meaningless clockwork motor which God or somebody installed 'at the beginning' and has run ever since. Life is no longer some menace that got into the perfect machine but is the creator of all. It is a living and conscious universe where energy and dynamic process are the basis of reality.

We now have a better and more functional model of health and disease. The age of energy medicine is here.
Dr Keith Scott-Mumby

Marbella 1999

FOREWORD

'Man cannot be completely seen, separate from mankind, nor mankind separate from all life, nor life separate from the Universe.'

Tielhard de Chardin, *Phenomena of Man*

There are books which are ahead of their time and books which do not break new ground in terms of recent intellectual developments. But, once in a while, a book like *Virtual Medicine* comes along which is truly pivotal. It seems to me that Keith Scott-Mumby is among the first to recognize the exact nature of the change which is taking place in the healing arts.

Scott-Mumby has managed to tread a careful path through the domain of esoteric, metaphysical matters, throwing light on the case and yet not being bogged down by the associated mystical rhetoric. His story reads like an 'adventure' into knowledge and is underpinned with frequent sound scientific references. In this way, Keith has pushed the cause of holism and integrated medicine considerably beyond its previous perameters.

Werner Heisenberg, one of the founders of modern quantum physics, said: *the most fruitful developments in human history have come when two different lines of thought have met.* Such 'lines' may have their roots in quite different parts of human culture, in different times, different intellectual environments and alien religions but they may nevertheless interact and produce new and exciting developments.

This seems to be the case with the Virtual Medicine paradigm. It is the meeting of Eastern philosophical healing systems and Western technological science which has led to a most fruitful advance which, as Keith remarks, is long overdue. Chinese and Ayurvedic models are based on the wisdom that the body possesses a natural ability to resist disease and heal itself, when correctly stimulated; only now are we able to work scientifically with these esoteric disciplines using new technology. And it is refreshing to note that, despite the preponderance of advanced scientific equipment, the unique bio-individuality of the patient is not lost. Otherwise, holistic medicine would simply go the way of its high-tech cousin.

One of Cowper's verses has led me to create a metaphor I would like to share:

Oars alone cannot prevail
To reach the distant coast,
The breath of Heaven must swell the sail,
Or else all toil is lost.

The oars, in this case, could be thought of as the Western electronic measuring and imaging systems explained by Keith. The breath of Heaven is surely the ancient and wonderfully vital energy of Eastern thinkers. The sail could be conceived as holistic man, as a mind-body-spirit conscious entity, which has been buffeted by the stormy winds of change in environment and lifestyle. These buffeting winds produce the stresses and toxins which shorten our lives. The coast, in turn, would be new dimensions of holistic and enlightened health for man.

Virtual Medicine both looks back over the ground we have conquered and forward with clarity and discernment into the future and where we are going. It is stimulating to the mind and intellect, well researched and written in accord with established medical parameters. I would wish to see it widely read, especially by our more conventional colleagues, and furthermore see this journey from metaphysics and philosophy to quantum physics and scientific realism adopted as tomorrows mainstream medical thinking and practise. Mankind is much in need of a gentler, more holistic technology in healing.

PROFESSOR (DR.MED) MICHAEL F. KIRKMAN
Chartered Biologist
Director Academic Affairs (GB), International Society of
Homotoxicology
External Advisor and Lecturer to the B.Sc(Hons) Course in Natural and
Complementary Medicine, University of Portsmouth

CHAPTER 1

JOIN THE PARTY, DOC

Our view of the world is changing fast. A quarter of a century ago there were things that scientists were absolutely *certain* were true which, today, we are absolutely certain are *not true*. Nowhere is this more evident than in the physics of organisms. In just a few decades we have moved from the position where the human energetic aura was deemed not to exist, to the point where there is ample scientific proof of its existence and several good theories as to its nature and function. Studies have been carried out in many major universities of the world which, although they are largely ignored by those who have some other 'truth' to peddle, have nevertheless done a great deal to unite realms that were once held to be only metaphysical (hence the name) with the accepted tenets of everyday science. We now have instruments which can measure effects on this order of reality; what is emerging is that the truth has indeed been out there a *long* time.

Nobody was really paying attention.

Until this recent era of enquiry into biological energy, any belief in the aura or psychokinetic effects was considered to be a childish construct of less scientific (and therefore mistaken) peoples; the typical view of our Western boffins was that what these peoples lacked in sophisticated understanding of reality they made up for in myths and 'mumbo-jumbo'. Shamans were just witch-doctors, and hands-on healing was a fraud that relied on self-delusion by gullible souls.

The mere fact that some of these supposedly naïve beliefs have been around for thousands of years, compared to a few centuries of our science, does not seem to carry any weight with those guilty of this hubris. Yet the reality is that science, as its own proponents define it, is a shifting quicksand of fashions and opinions, which regularly contradicts itself – often embarrassingly so. Two of the grandest and most revolutionary theories of this century, Einstein's Relativity and Planck's Quantum mechanics, are in such disharmony that they appear mutually exclusive. The Big Bang hypothesis of cosmology has all but collapsed due to inconsistencies, according to Professor Andrei Linde at California's Stanford University, though those who make their living writing about it refuse to admit there are major discrepancies, and march on blindly as if nothing were wrong.[1] It is a disconcerting fact that electricity and magnetism, two of the absolutely fundamental building blocks of the universe, are so little understood that, at the deepest level, science cannot explain the nature of these energetic phenomena or how they exert their effect. We recognize the electron as a basic building block, which has properties such as mass and charge, but a deeper explanation of how these properties arise is lacking.

I make this point in case the reader is under the illusion that science, in any meaningful sense, understands our world. It doesn't.

My greatest complaint with so-called science is that it fails to acknowledge that whenever something cannot be shown to exist using the standard approach, it is labelled 'unscientific' and therefore a fake or delusion. There is never any suggestion that the problem may be the fault of science or its inadequate methodology. Yet 100 years ago there was no way to detect radio waves. Did that mean they were an 'unscientific' belief, if anyone had come up with the idea ahead of its time? Even more importantly, could it be said that because the science of the day failed to detect such a phenomenon *that therefore radio waves did not exist?*

THE REBIRTH OF VITALISM

Philosophers speak of an epistemology of 'naïve realism'; it means thinking that all you see is all there is. Very naïve.

Yet modern mechanistic science is stuck in this frame of mind. It is predicated wholly on the belief that there is nothing more to our experience of Being than a heap of matter which (supposedly) came into existence ready-formed in some giant flash at the start of time. The irony of this is that Isaac Newton, who fathered this view of the world, was himself deeply embroiled in the occult, magic, alchemy and other mystical matters which today's scientist effects to despise and ridicule. Of course it is Newton's followers who have gone over the edge into the legitimacy of this so-called 'clockwork' universe. The dismay of his biographers in trying to reconcile the man as they wanted to see him and the truth of his past led to the virtual suppression of most of his writings – 'The obvious production of a fool and a knave,' as one of his biographers described this secret material.[2]

In the 20th century we have been forced to look again at the mechanistic universe and, finally, brave new writers like Rupert Sheldrake are coming out with a refreshing paradigm, which is that life and the conscious process make matter, and not the other way round.[3] The model of the world in which the energies of life are pre-eminent and drive creation is called *Vitalism*. One of the greatest proponents of this philosophy was Henri Bergson (1859–1941), who received the Nobel Prize for literature in 1927 and became a member of l'Académie Française (1941). He is author of *Matter and Memory* (1896) and *Creative Evolution* (1907). Sir John C. Eccles, (1903–) the distinguished Australian neurophysiologist and 1963 Nobel laureate, expounds his version of Vitalism in *Evolution of the Brain: Creation of the Self*.[4] Vitalism is the traditional view of the world, eclipsed briefly for a few centuries under the weight of scientific excesses, but now forcing itself upon us as the only truth which can explain what we see – no fudging.

Of course it would be wrong to try and remove the word 'science' from the dictionary of common-sense. But science needs rehabilitating from the pompous and pedantic position it has taken and made into what it should be: the discipline of knowledge and learning *all the truth*. In the fullest sense, science, philosophy and religion come together. There can be no science that violates the precepts of sacredness and Being, attempting to dismiss life as some weird accident in the chemical machine.

INFORMATION FIELDS

The newest concept in biology is the *information field*. Information fields create reality; they put it there and hold it together the way it should be. Have you ever wondered why a teacup is a teacup? Why don't the atoms at the edge go wandering off and become, say, a spoon? The answer is an information field. When you drink a cup of tea you do so from something which, in material terms, is 99.999999 per cent not there (please don't count the decimal places, there are dozens I didn't bother to type). Only the field is real. Matter, as quantum physics teaches us, is a mere illusion. It comes out of this 'void' or vacuum, whenever we interact with it. Like the cavalry troops in the old B movies, it shows up just when it's needed!

It follows that a cancer, a parasite or a virus are also just information fields. Everything in our life and being is energy and information. We come from fields in the egg; we go back to a field as a corpse. Indeed, there is the likelihood that we survive death at least as some kind of field.

Biological information fields are unbelievably vast in the amount of data which they contain — many orders of magnitude greater than the combined total molecular complexity of our physical substances. In other words, there is no way that the bio-chemical plasma of our bodies could contain enough information to organize and control a living organism. We need the information field to put us there and hold us in place. Chemicals cannot 'think' and organize other chemicals without some initiating input! This one fact really does put paid once and for all to the idea of biochemically-based life, as espoused by the current drug-based medical culture. We exist as regulated and informed energy.

According to 1984 Nobel Laureate Carlo Rubbia, matter ('stuff') is less than a billionth part of the manifest cosmos. The rest is pure energy phenomena of interaction, information fields and resonance. This is a staggering revelation, from one of science's top minds. A healing discipline which looks only at such a tiny and inconsequential part of the whole is badly skewed, and is bound to get it wrong more often than right. Stuck in the incorrect 'matter' paradigm, ignorant doctors are surely doomed to violate the first precept of Hippocrates' code, which is: 'Do no harm.'

Unfortunately, doctors are decades behind with this and are not even talking about the idea yet. Scientific attitudes here, I am sorry to say, are often no more than an affectation with which the medical establishment tries to brow-beat its (many) opponents, rather than the humble reality of willing seekers of truth. It is a case where, as the founder of humanistic psychology Abram Maslow put it, the pretence of science is being used to avoid the bigger truth.

FIELD DISTURBANCES

Remember that information implies consciousness of a sort. It is inescapable. David Pearson, with his theories of the 'living universe' (conscious matter), has found remarkable success and accord among physics and mathematical colleagues. But once again the doctors were not at the party![5]

It is interesting to note that the word information means to give material form to (from the Latin: *informare*). In other words, information at the quantum field level is actually an active, creative force intimately involved in the form and manifestation of reality. Stated differently, information is a specific way of representing the interaction of consciousness and reality, either as a means of organizing it or decoding it. It is too early to be sure *how* these fields operate and influence things, except to say that quantum probability fields seem the intermediate domain between consciousness and reality made manifest. Even without a full understanding, it is a major paradigm shift to recognize they are there and the critical role they play.

Disease can now be redefined as a disruption, cessation or distortion arising in the information and energy fields. The *best* way to approach disease then, surely, is by correcting these disturbances, which will then eliminate the disharmony and disease process – in other words, bring about healing.

We call this **Energy Medicine** (sometimes vibrational medicine) and it is a theme which is central to the material in this book. If virtual reality means virtual fields, and virtual matter springs from virtual energy, then it's time we gave up the whole idea of the importance of material substances and started to think differently about our world. As soon as we do so, the world begins to take on a spiritual, almost metaphysical reality, and religious factors enter into the equation. As Dr Richard Gerber, author of *Vibrational Medicine*, says, 'The unseen connection between the physical body and the subtle forces of spirit holds the key to understanding the inner relationship between matter and energy. When scientists begin to comprehend the true relationship between matter and energy, they will come closer to understanding the relationship between humanity and God.'[6]

Healing, then, becomes a loving matter of bringing to the distressed part or organism some kindly or enfolding energy or resonance which soothes the disharmony and coaxes forth healing, instead of violently suppressing the symptoms, which are only manifestations of the body's 'fight-back' response. This healing method is both more rational and more effective, since manifestly we are going further 'upstream' to treat and cure. In fact if we go far enough towards the source, we inevitably encounter the mystery and might of consciousness itself.

The role of consciousness in health and disease has yet to be grasped by the average physician, but it is impossible to leave it to mystics and theological scholars. The nature of life and Being is the key to the door of healing! I believe consciousness is a kind of creative energy force and that, whether we understand it or not, we need to try and work towards incorporating it in our model of health and disease. Life is an expression of this consciousness, as the shamans have been telling us.

DULL TUMMY, NOT SO DULL RESEARCH

At the start of this century, distinguished American neurologist Albert Abrams observed something remarkable, though for all his life he was totally unable to explain it. The man was no intellectual lightweight and had studied conventional medicine with the best doctors of the time in Europe – Virchow, Wasserman, Helmholz and others – winning top honours and a gold medal from Heidelberg University. You can be sure he knew what he was seeing, even if he couldn't understand it.

Abrams returned to the US and taught pathology at Stanford University's medical school in California. One day, when he was percussing (tapping on) the abdomen of a patient with his fingers, the resonant note went suddenly dull. It coincided with the moment when a nearby x-ray machine was switched on. But what was remarkable was that when Abrams rotated the patient, he found the dull note was only present when the patient was oriented east—west. It was a spectacular example of science from a serendipitous moment, where the prepared mind, in the right place at the right time, observes something which everyone else would surely miss.

Subsequently, during a routine examination of a patient suffering from cancer (of the lip), Abrams noticed the same strange dull percussion note when tapping certain areas of the abdomen. It turned up on other cancer patients and tuberculosis cases, but again only if the body was aligned with feet towards the west. Abrams subsequently found this dullness in healthy cases when they were merely in close proximity to cancer or tuberculosis specimens and, most astonishing of all, in cases where the patient was remote from the pathological disease specimen but connected to it by means of a wire.[7]

Abrams' conclusion, quite logically, was that unknown waves were being emitted by diseased tissue and that these could produce physical alteration within the body. He went on to find that he could pass a metal disc over the patient's body, connected to the wire, and when he came to the site of pathology the note would again go dull. When a sceptical colleague challenged him to find the exact location of a tuberculous infection of the lung, Abrams did so accurately. He was able to repeat this numerous times in different cases and with uncanny accuracy.

Abrams went on to develop an instrument he called the *Reflexophone* as a means of detecting and quantifying the strange radiation. A variable resistance altered the current and the machine emitted a sound which varied in pitch, thus eliminating the need to percuss the abdomen. He spoke in terms of differing 'rates' for each disease process and compiled a disease register: 55 for syphilis, 58 for sarcomatous tissue, and so on. Even when testing blind, he could infallibly detect or 'diagnose' disease tissue, using his device. Even more incredibly, Abrams found that by adding new resistors to the Reflexophone, he could calibrate the device in such a way it would say how far advanced the disease process was! Finally, as if to annoy his conventional colleagues to the extreme, Abrams announced that he could dispense with the patient's physical presence altogether and use only a spot of the subject's blood, hair or urine for testing. Not only that, but he could obtain his 'electronic reactions' by having a healthy subject point to the part of their own body which was diseased in the patient, while connected to the Reflexophone. It was all too fantastic to believe.

One day, while Abrams was demonstrating to a class the reaction produced by the blood of a malaria patient, he went one stage further. The known treatment of malaria was quinine, an alkaloid from the bark of the Cinchona tree. Abrams put a few grains of quinine sulphate into the test tray, together with the malarial blood and, to everyone's amazement, the dull percussion note vanished. The reaction was cancelled out. Other known antidotes behaved similarly; for example, mercurial salts for syphilis. With the insight of genius, Abrams suggested there were unknown radiations emitted by the quinine molecule which *exactly* cancelled out the emanations from the malaria specimen.

From this he reasoned, logically, that it should be possible to build a machine which could broadcast electrical oscillations at just the right counter-frequency, and thereby alter the characteristics of diseased tissue and effect a cure. In co-operation with Samuel O. Hoffman, a radio research engineer who had distinguished himself in the First World War by devising an early form of radar to detect approaching German zeppelins at a great distance, Abrams came up with his *Oscilloclast*. It did indeed offer some remarkable cures. His ideas began to spread and shake the foundations of the medical establishment. In his prophetic words, 'As physicians we dare not stand aloof from the progress made in physical science and segregate the human entity from other entities of the physical universe.'

However, conventional science was not ready for this new wisdom.

Predictably, Abrams was attacked and vilified. When he perhaps unwisely announced in 1922 that he had used his instruments to successfully diagnose a patient over telephone wires, he was quickly denounced as a quack in the *Journal of the American Medical Association*. When the *British Medical Journal* repeated the scurrilous and defamatory attack, Sir James Barr, past president of the British Medical Association, wrote furiously in defence of Abrams: 'You [BMJ] very seldom quote from the *Journal of the American Medical Association* and one might have expected that when you did you would have chosen a more serious subject than an ignorant tirade against an eminent medical man, against, in my opinion, the greatest genius in the medical profession.' Barr went on to gibe that, one day, 'medical editors and medical men will begin to perceive that there was more to Abrams' vibrations than was dreamt of in their philosophy.'

Abrams died in 1924. The vituperation continued for some time, including 18 consecutive issues of *Scientific American*. One of the worst insinuations was that Abrams had no scientific motive but was merely trying to make money by gulling an unsuspecting community. In truth, Abrams, son of a rich San Francisco merchant, had inherited a vast fortune and was a millionaire in his own right. He had written to Upton Sinclair, the American writer and journalist, offering to donate his devices and work *unpaid* for any institute which would develop the 'Abrams Box' for the benefit of humanity.

Such is the integrity of medical journalism.

I can testify personally. Though no innovative genius, I followed in the footsteps of this remarkable man, proud to do so, when I was denounced by the *British Medical Journal* in 1993 as a clinical ecology charlatan. Apart from flirting with journalists, I was basically accused of misleading people with the absurd idea that their diet and environment could make them ill and that this could be prevented. A certain Professor Barry Kay was allowed to repeat defamatory allegations which I had defended fully and been acquitted of before a disciplinary tribunal, on the intellectually specious grounds that I *should* have been found guilty! But a firm word from my libel lawyer, and in this happy instance I was allowed to write my own extended response, which I did under the title *'Science or Flat Earthers!'*[8] All I stood for has subsequently been established in scientific literature.

THE EMANOMETER

There is another twist to the enthralling story, in which the truth fared a little better. It is worth telling in brief, since it is important to the credibility of the Virtual Medicine paradigm. In 1922 a British homeopathic physician, Dr William Boyd, built a modified version of the Oscilloclast called an Emanometer, and confirmed all Abrams' findings. Boyd was a keen researcher, particularly in the field of electro-physics, and he published extensive scientific physiological and biochemical research. He presented a very detailed paper on the workings of the Emanometer at the International Homeopathic Conference in London in 1927. As well as diagnosing, Boyd used it to test homeopathic remedies and let the instrument choose a suitable similimum (for a full account of homeopathy and Virtual Medicine, see Chapter 7). It was quite successful by all accounts — but it was all so startling that controversy was, of course, inevitable.

Accordingly, in 1924 a committee was set up by the Royal Society of Medicine to investigate Boyd's claims, under the chairmanship of Sir Thomas Horder (later Lord Horder). The results were reported to the Royal Society of Medicine in January 1925. It is little short of astonishing that Horder found the Emanometer and percussion method quite valid; over the space of years I pay respect to his integrity. One would have expected official fudging. The fact is, all the committee members were able to detect the change in percussion note first described by Abrams, and the detector apparatus was considered to offer important new diagnostic possibilities. In a series of 25 trials, Boyd's method was shown to be 100 per cent accurate, identifying chemicals and tissues presented in a manner which was 'indistinguishable by visual or other normal' means.[9]

However, the committee made no cogent recommendations

for further research, and since neither they nor Boyd had the faintest idea how the equipment might work, the Black Box was subsequently ignored and passed into medical history. It now stands as a watchword for humbug and pseudo-science among the sceptics. However, this story is far from ended, as later chapters on electro-acupuncture and electro-dermal screening with a modern computer will reveal.

Meanwhile, George de la Warr in Britain and Ruth Drown in the US had devised their own versions of Abrams' instrument, and for a time considerable interest began to develop in radiesthesia or radionics, as their new technique became known. However, the enthusiasts were to remain entirely outside the medical profession and detector instruments were soon being sold to all and sundry, most of whom had no legal medical qualifications. Inevitably bizarre, exaggerated or just stupid interpretations were being made which soon brought the whole system into grave disrepute.

The catastrophic and manifestly unjust imprisonment of Ruth Drown for supposed fraud shattered any remaining credibility and heralded the end of any chance for the new medicine to slip into mainstream practice (she had been tricked by use of a spot of chicken blood on which she had passed a 'diagnosis'). Radionics limps on, staunchly defended by a few nobly-indignant devotees but hardly taken seriously, even by most fringe practitioners. It has been unable to shake off the stigma of its shaky beginnings and the criminal indictment of its principal founder.

BIOLOGICAL RESONANCE

The key question here is: 'What scientific effect had Abrams found?' It might be argued that one or two paid practitioners were fraudsters; but members of a UK Government committee were hardly likely all to be stooges. They had seen *something* credible, after all. Can we put a name to it after all this time? I believe the answer is an unqualified 'Yes', and it is not magic moonbeams or alien rays.

Abrams himself discovered a clue. While he was in Naples he watched the famous tenor Enrico Caruso flick a wine glass to produce its note or tone and then, by singing the same note, shatter the glass. We call this phenomenon *resonance*. You can try it for yourself in the bathtub; simply sing or hum a higher and higher note and at some point you will hear a loud booming effect where the loudness of the sound is markedly enhanced. At this exact pitch your voice is resonating with the basic wavelength of the room, according to its size (the smaller the room, the higher the resonance note).

In my view, the so-called Abrams' reflex was a spectacular example of the principle of *cyclotron resonance*, though demonstrated over half a century before this important magnetic phenomenon was recognized and explained. With the discovery of the cyclotron resonance effect, advanced physics is almost ready to shake hands with energy healing and telepathy. It is critical to the understanding of the functioning of most of the remarkable new diagnostic and therapy systems in the chapters which follow.

Nobel Prize double-nominee Robert O. Becker tells us, 'The electromagnetic resonance concept may provide an intriguing link to a number of little understood and disputed phenomena, such as extrasensory perception and the ability of "healers" to diagnose and treat patients. In both these activities, the participants may be unconsciously using an innate biological mechanism similar to that of magnetic-resonance imaging (MRI).'[10]

Everyone today is familiar with MRI, though usually without necessarily comprehending the technicalities involved. In principle it isn't difficult, though of course the reality may be far more involved than we know. A charged particle or chemical 'ion', when in a fixed magnetic field such as the earth's own field, is made to spin; the stronger the magnetic effect, the faster the spin. Each atomic substance has different spin characteristics.

If a second oscillating (ON—OFF) field is applied, at an angle of (exactly) 90 degrees to the original field, then the spin motion is enhanced according to the principle we call resonance; it is the same effect as piano or violin strings beginning to hum in sympathy with musical notes of the right frequency sounded nearby. The particles *gain* energy. If the field is suddenly interrupted, the particles give up this extra energy, which is radiated outwards (Figure 1). An image can be formed by placing the body in a fixed field and then bombarding it with an oscillating field, flowing at right angles. When the oscillating field is ON, the ions pick up energy; when the oscillating field is OFF, the ions re-radiate the energy in a form which can be picked up and displayed on a computer as a three-dimensional image. That's really all there is to MRI.

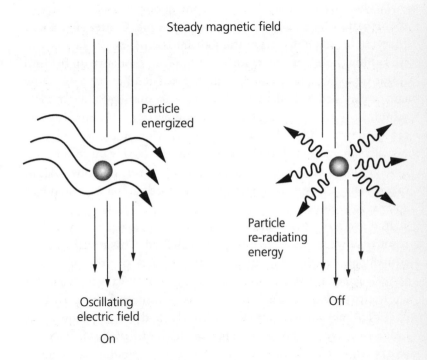

The enhanced energy effect we call cyclotron resonance. What is important is that the weaker the static field, the smaller the oscillating cross-field needed to create the resonance effect.

It is impossible to over-estimate the biological importance of this. Living forms exist within the Earth's field, which is very weak. Thus only the slightest disturbance, if at the right frequency and in the critical direction, could have profound effects on important ions such as calcium, sodium and potassium (note how Abrams' reflex *only* operated if the body was oriented feet to the West). It is only a matter of time before scientists begin to wonder if certain diseases are not becoming more common because the typical fields we experience are the ones which interfere with the ordered metabolism of critical ions (the rise in osteoporosis, which depends on functioning levels of calcium ions, is an example I have in mind). So far as I know, no-one has yet shared this type of speculation. You read it here first!

To show how easily this could come about, consider an experiment carried out at the US Naval Research Center, Bethesda, Maryland, and published in the journal *Biomagnetics* in 1986. In this study the effects of cyclotron magnetic resonance on lithium in rat brains was monitored, using a fixed field of 0.2 gauss (low end of the Earth's field strength) and an oscillating field of 60 Hz, which is the frequency of the US domestic mains supply. The reasoning was that if the lithium was truly enhanced by the magnetic resonance effect, then the rats should display more subdued behaviour, since lithium is known as a central nervous system depressant. Unexposed controls were used, as part of standard scientific protocol.[11]

In due course, it was obvious that the rats exposed to cyclotron resonance were indeed significantly subdued. This result was the equivalent of giving the rats a substantial dose of lithium; in fact they had been given none. The study is important because it shows major biological effects with low-strength fields acting on chemical substances common within the body. It also shows that fields in a typical home are significant biologically. In fact we worry a great deal these days about the particular frequencies between 10 and 100 Hz. These are considered extremely-low-frequency, or ELF, fields. The US military is seeking to develop weapons and population control using this type of radiation. It may be less destructive than nuclear warfare, but such abuse of scientific knowledge is reprehensible and very sinister (see page 182).

RESONANCE IN THE HEALING CONTEXT

You may be sure that the military does not involve itself in phenomena which are illusory (other than the general case of trying to 'win' a war by killing people and destroying material goods). On the contrary, the military is often responsible for important new advances in technology, such as radar, jet engines and space rockets. In time, these new concepts in the physical sciences will filter into the medical model, bypassing the Galenite die-hards, and create what will surely be a major paradigm shift. Hopefully, research will rapidly advance and what many practising therapists from a number of holistic disciplines have known for years will be found to have a credible scientific footing. It is a constant lament of mine that if only doctors knew more advanced physics, they would be less inclined to attack alternative healing. Experiments using the newest scientific test devices, such as the SQUID magnetometer (see Chapter 2), have shown conclusively that hands-on healers are able to generate a magnetic field around their hands. Indeed, a skilled healer merges his or her whole body field with that of the patient. It is entirely possible, indeed probable, that these healers interact on the resonance principle and create effects which, though we do not understand them properly, begin to fit with known measured reality.

Even 'faith healing' may not be a matter of faith, after all.

ENERGY BEING

We have now reached the stage where we can sensibly postulate life as an energy Being which is manifest in the presence of a body or organism but is definitely *not* confined to the physical structure concerned. This energy presence is a source for wholesome good in the organism but may, due to various reasons yet little understood, become corrupted or disturbed and so give off harmful emanations which act upon the body organism and result in the disease process. The way is open for many legitimate healing techniques which can diagnose using these energy changes, and cause beneficial modifications of the energy forces. I have termed this concept **Virtual Medicine**, since nothing is done in the material domain. Only the results are felt there.

Everything takes place in a super-ordinate world of information and energy.

What has stimulated this book is the recognition that the world of high-tech medicine and cutting-edge physics is beginning to drift markedly in the direction of alternative development streams in healing. There is equipment we shall be reviewing which has been around even longer than CAT scanners and MRI, which can tell us a great deal about the health and biological status of a human being. In the chapters to follow we will be looking at systems which can:

- 'listen' for the transmission of rabies from the tissues
- tell from the distressed energies which is the most disturbed organ of the body
- detect old and unresolved diseases which can affect our present health
- tell electronically whether disease is psychosomatic
- sense the development of cancer as an energy field *years* before it actually becomes manifest as a disease entity.

We are entering a totally new world-view where electronics, quantum physics and the computer meet age-old wisdom of the mind and body. It is time for medical practitioners to join the party.

CHAPTER 2

THE HISTORY OF ENERGY MEDICINE

The energy-based medicine paradigm has been a very long time in coming. In various forms it goes back to the depths of time and was (and still is) practised by shamans. The ancient Egyptians had a version of hands-on healing; the Ebers papyrus urges: 'Lay your hands on him to ease his pain and order his suffering to disappear.' It is entirely possible that the Bible stories of Jesus healing people recount a form of beneficial energy transfer.

HANDS-ON HEALING

Schiegl also describes the technique of *shunomatism*, named after a woman known as Abisag from Shuna who slept with King David to bring him back to health.[1] The concept of lying down with someone ill in order to take on their evil humours is told of in other tales as well. According to one story, Lady Bath of England slept with two young women; she recovered and they were left drained and ill. One might imagine other explanations for this type of recovery, but it is entirely consistent with Tantric teachings of energy transference.

PARACELSUS

The great Middle Age physician who called himself Paracelsus (Theophrastus Philippus Bombastus von Hohenheim) expostulated theories of health and disease based on an astral fluid, which we may liken to a bio-energy field and which he called *archea*. His method hypothesized sucking out the ill-humours or negative energy. He wrote about Earth magnetism, and readily spotted it had enormous power to influence our lives. In every way he was a visionary and brilliant man, centuries ahead of his time and someone who is still revered, and rightly so, by all practitioners of holistic and spiritually-oriented therapies. His major tract *De Origine Morborum Invisibilum* (*The Invisible Causes of Diseases*) nicely presages the title for my own present work! He would be pleased to see the revelations that science offers true-healing medicine described in this book.

ANTON MESMER

The other great figure who must be introduced in any review like this is Anton Mesmer. Born in 1734, he properly belongs to the modern scientific (post-Newton) age. Few figures have ever made such an impression on their era, or paid so dearly for assaulting the vagaries of medical orthodoxy. Even today his name is synonymous with smoke-and-mirrors mystification – to 'mesmerize' someone often means to somehow overthrow their common sense and harness their credulity. Yet this is to woefully misinterpret Mesmer's work.

Mesmer took some of his inspiration from earlier thinkers, including Paracelsus. He worked on energetic healing using systematic movements of the hands. Judging by the enormous numbers of people who came to him, he must have been very successful. He recognized a healing force of some kind coming through his hands; he even found he could transfer it indirectly through other individuals. He invented the term 'animal magnetism'. Unfortunately there was no way in his day to measure such a force field and he was ultimately discredited. Yet he was right, as we shall see. Today, just before the close of the 20th century, we are able to visualize the energies that he could sense and describe.

In Mesmer's work *Report on the Discovery of Animal Magnetism* he describes 27 axiomatic principles, which many enlightened doctors today would consider to remain valid. Only the terminology has changed. Here are a few of these key principles:

1 There is a mutual influence of celestial bodies, the Earth and human bodies [see 'the peculiar properties of water', page 110].

2 The medium for this influence is a universally present and continuous fluid, which permeates everywhere. It is

fine beyond comparison, and by its nature, is capable of receiving, spreading and communicating all influences of movement [the quantum field].

3 The mutual influence is subject to laws of mechanics that are as yet unknown [quantum mechanics].

4 The living body feels the alternative effects of this fluid: by penetrating the nerves, these are directly affected [neuro-peptide release; current model for much successful therapy].

Again, Mesmer was a man far ahead of his time and we have to move to the 20th century for further significant advances.

FIELDS OF LIFE

In the 1920s and 1930s Professor Harold Saxton Burr at Yale University began to experiment with electrical recordings of living energy fields of trees and, subsequently, humans. Trees were particularly suitable since they could be left wired up for long periods. Burr was fascinated to note changes brought about by sunlight and darkness, cycles of the moon, sunspots and seasonal changes.

Studying humans, he and his colleague Dr Leonard Ravitz noticed that human emotions affected this field. Voltages would be high when a patient was feeling good and would drop when he or she was below par. Burr foresaw the fascinating possibility that '... psychiatrists of the future will be able to measure the intensity of grief, anger or love electrically — as easily as we now measure temperature or noise-levels today. "Heartbreak", hate or love, in other words, may one day be measurable in millivolts.'[2]

Burr and colleagues also discovered a voltage rise just before ovulation, which drops just as the egg is released. Healing wounds also changed this voltage. Most remarkable of all, there were voltage changes due to malignant tissue and Burr was eventually able to predict, from reversal of the polarity across the abdominal wall, when a woman would in future develop cancer of the cervix.[3] This anticipates later prognostic work with electro-dermal screening described in Chapter 8.

What Burr and his colleagues were measuring was simply voltage potential. But he himself points out that changes can be measured at a distance from the affected organ or even outside the body, holding the electrodes above the skin, showing it is therefore a true field effect. He called it the 'Field of Life', or L-Field for short.

LAKHOVSKY

The next investigative genius was actually born in 1869; his seminal book *The Secret of Life* was published in 1925. This puts him ahead (chronologically) of Saxton Burr, but the reader will soon readily appreciate that progressively he belongs here in the sequence, since his visionary ideas look far forward into the world of modern bio-physics.

Georges Lakhovsky was a Russian engineer who became a naturalized French citizen and was ultimately awarded the Legion of Honour for his scientific technical services during the First World War. He had to flee his adopted country before the arrival of the Nazis, and died in New York in 1942.

Like those who went before him, Lakhovsky had to endure much calumny and ridicule. As one of his supporters remarked: 'The publication of *The Secret of Life* resulted in causing great annoyance to the custodians of infallible doctrines who made up with carping verbiage what they lacked in clarity of vision.'[4] As Lakhovsky himself put it: 'I have been attacked by physicists ignorant of biology and by biologists ignorant of physics who consequently can neither understand my theories nor judge my experiments.'[5] This extraordinary man of diverse talents showed that recorded sunspot activity parallelled magnetic disturbances and auroras on Earth. He also established a correlation between sunspot activity and good wine vintage years. In my own book *The Complete Guide to Food Allergy and Environmental Illness* I call attention to Lakhovsky's observation that geological terrain seems to have a potentially dangerous connection with cancer causation.[6] Clay soils in particular, he found, were dangerous, probably because of the properties of water within the soil, whereas sandy and limestone soils had a very much lower incidence of carcinogenisis. Lakhovsky also foresaw that one day it might be possible to project images of cancer tumours as an energy disturbance onto a TV screen; today we have MRI and CAT scanners.

But it is Lakhovsky's ideas about biological radiation fields that concern us here. His fundamental scientific principle was that *every living thing emits radiation*. This has important health implications. According to Lakhovsky, the nucleus of a living cell may be compared to an electrical oscillating circuit. This nucleus consists of tubular filaments, chromosomes and mitochondria, made of insulating membranes but filled by an electrically-conductive intra-cellular fluid. These filaments have capacitance and inductance properties and are therefore capable of working like radio transmitters and receivers.

Some time ago, UK research scientist Roger Coghill extended Lakhovsky's insight by suggesting that the DNA molecule is the ideal shape (a spiral) for a radio-transmitting aerial. Perhaps the morphogenic field that tells an organism how to grow from its genes may in fact be an energy-message radioed from the DNA 'radio station'! (Coghill now considers it more likely to be the glyco-proteins – sugary molecules which stand up from the cell surface – which act like little aerials.)

In Lakhovsky's model, life and disease are a matter of a 'war of radiations' between the body's cells and microbes. If the radiations of the microbe win, disease and death will result. If the cell's own energy transmission wins, then health is preserved. Thus he arrived at a very advanced and quite defensible energetic view of disease. Lakhovsky himself went on to conduct very many experiments in this vein. The results he got were little short of startling for his time, and so one may presume there is a lot to be derived from his theories.

Albert Nodon, President of the Société Astronomique of Bordeaux, studying ultra-short waves in organisms, was able to prove Lakhovsky's hypothesis. He found radiation from all living plants and animals. Dead subjects did not, of course, transmit. Nodon produced remarkable figures showing that, weight for weight, radiation from certain beetles, flies and spiders was 3 to 15 times more intense than that from uranium. He extended his studies to humans and was able to show that our bodies emit even more intense energies than plants and animals. Nodon also obtained what were termed 'spontaneous radiographs' by placing living things directly onto photographic plates. Clear pictures were duly developed, after several hours exposure. This forgotten research anticipated Kirlian photography by many decades. Nodon's conclusion was 'It seems probable that matter, under the influence of radiation whose wavelength is less than the electron, may be subjected to certain modifications of an unknown nature which may confer new properties on matter, different from those conferred by radiations of a much greater wavelength, and not connected with electrons.'[7]

How right he was all those years ago.

For many years Lakhovsky had a great interest in the mechanism of cancer-formation. This in itself was unusual in his time. There were no 'Fight Cancer' media campaigns running then, and a leading London surgeon of the day pointed out that funding of cancer research did not even amount to one penny per person in the British Isles!

There have been many hypotheses advanced as to the causation of this pathological blight, including heredity, infection by viruses, local trauma, pollution and nutritional deficiency. It seems probable that all these factors may play a part. But Lakhovsky was convinced that oscillatory disequilibrium – that is, cellular radiation energy disturbance – was the predominant factor in the onset of malignancy.

The problem was, how to reverse it.

Our bodies consist of some 200,000,000,000,000,000,000 cells, and hardly any two oscillate exactly alike. This is partly due to differing tissues but also variation through time in the status of each individual cell. The impact of extraneous radiation would also produce modulations, such as the resonance effect. Finding a standardized harmonizing frequency would seem to be a Sisyphean task.

With brilliance and ingenuity, Lakhovsky invented his celebrated Multiple Wave Oscillator, generating a field in which every cell could find its own frequency and vibrate in resonance. The practical successes he began having in hospitals soon confirmed the validity of his theory. Numerous cases recovered and were documented by excited doctors.

Lakhovsky was careful to avoid talking in terms of a cancer 'cure'; however he did unequivocally cure a number of cases, and all the others showed variable but marked degrees of improvement.

If any reader would like to follow one of his simple experiments on plant cancer, it is not difficult to perform and will provide a fascinating home workshop on the properties of biological radiation. In this experiment Lakhovsky purposely dispensed with the oscillator and relied instead on the presence of ambient radiations. He took a series of Geranium plants inoculated with the Bacterium tumefaciens (= tumour-making) which causes cancer-like growths on the plants:

A month later, when the tumours had developed, I took one of the plants at random which I surrounded with a spiral consisting of copper and measuring 30 cm in diameter, its two extremities, not joined together, being fixed into an ebonite support [a rigid plastic tube, such as a spent biro pen stem, would suffice perfectly well]. An oscillator of this kind has a fundamental wavelength of about 2 metres (150 million Hcrz) and picks up the oscillating energy of innumerable radiations in the atmosphere.

I then let the experiment follow its natural course during several weeks. After a fortnight, I examined my plants. I was astonished to find that all my geraniums or the stalks bearing the tumours were dead and dried up with the exception of the geranium surrounded by the copper spiral, which has since grown to twice the height of the untreated healthy plants.[8]

The oscillator was picking up and damping all kinds of atmospheric radiations. Lakhovsky bewailed the fact that so many radio transmitters were springing up (even in his day) that 'there is no detectable gap in the gamut of these waves'. Consider the health problem implied by this, when today we have a million times the intensity of blanket radiations that he experienced.

We will discuss this further in Chapter 10.

DR GEORGE CRILE

Famous US surgeon George Crile, founder of the celebrated Cleveland Clinic in Ohio, published almost contemporaneously with Lakhovsky, and their theories and predictions bear striking resemblances. I have chosen Lakhovsky mainly because, in my opinion, he was the more visionary of the two. Crile's radical work *The Phenomena of Life – A Radio-electric Interpretation* shows that he may be said to have discovered independently the same facts as Lakhovsky and used the same theories to explain his observation.

Addressing a congress of the American College of Surgeons in Chicago, October 1933, Crile pointed out that as the fundamental sciences of physics and chemistry advance their knowledge it should be possible in the future for the skilled radio-diagnosti-cian to detect the presence of disease before it becomes apparent. If you want to know just how accurate this prediction is and can-not wait, turn to Chapter 8.

Crile foresaw Virtual Medicine.

THE SALAMANDER MAN

Enter Professor Robert Becker, orthopaedic surgeon and twice-Nobel Prize nominee. He is the first person on this list of pio-neers and visionaries who is still alive today and making his views felt. He is noted especially for research into biological elec-trical potentials, but has gone on to become the doyen of energy medicine and the darling of the New Agers who, judging by fuss-ings on the Internet, are looking for some scientific credence for their treasured mystical views.

However Becker is not to be much distracted by celebrity sta-tus and one can tell from his writings that he views being embraced by the alternative medicine movement with some alarm. He carefully distances himself from anything which does-n't fall into the strictest scientific rhetoric.

From years of experimental work on salamanders, showing that living organisms propagate a DC electrical field and that this undergoes certain changes when the salamanders are diseased and injured (exactly what Burr showed), Becker has developed elegant new theories regarding the electromagnetic regulation of life processes.[9] But Becker has gone further, with more advanced measuring systems, and has been able to show that body tissues act as semi-conductors, and that this is how the life-currents are transmitted. I find this exciting because it implies the possibility that living cells and tissues can function in the manner of a com-puter, providing there is suitable software (not that I think life is computer-modelled). So far, in my studies for this book I have not found anyone, not even Becker himself, who has had the same speculative thought.

Becker also showed, in his research into the subject of de-differentiation, that cells reverting to more primitive grades in response to stress (which is supposed to be impossible according to modern theories) not only takes place but can be deliberately provoked in frog red blood cells by a very tiny current which he measured in billionths of an ampere. Even a slightly stronger current did not have the desired effect, which would surprise the modern scientific community but not alternative practitioners, who have long understood the precept of gently coaxing a response from Nature rather than blasting it into action (which usually doesn't work). What Becker discovered is a version of the Arndt-Schulz low-dose homeopathic law given in full on page 120.

In the 1970s Becker and his biophysicist colleague, Maria Reichmanis, were funded by the US National Institutes of Health to study acupuncture scientifically. He chose to measure DC potential (electricity given off) at designated acupuncture points, and claims to have found that around 25 per cent of the points on the forearm were locatable using this method. He also showed that current is conducted by unknown channels which correspond to the stated acupuncture meridians. It is worth pointing out here that later in the book I will discuss research using changes in skin resistance at acupuncture points, which may be a more accurate method of detection. Proof of the probable nature of acupuncture meridians follows in Chapter 3.

Over the years Becker has expanded his authority and knowledge to be considered one of the best-informed scientists on the big issues of bio-physics and environmental hazards, particularly those concerning the effects of electric and magnetic fields on living systems. His recent book *Cross Currents: The Perils of Electropollution; The Promise of Electromedicine* is an extremely powerfully argued and comprehensive overview of what has been going on in the last two decades in the field of electro-biology. He didn't coin the term energy medicine, but he has certainly given it life breath and lifted it into the domain of science.

I particularly like his classification of energy medicine into three categories, according to the force used:

1 Minimal Energy Techniques: No actual physical energy transferred. Examples would include creative visualization or hypnosis.

2 Energy-reinforcement Techniques: Adding to and supporting the body's natural energies. He cited acupuncture
and homeopathy.

3 High-energy Transfer Techniques: supplying energy at
higher-than-natural levels. Examples would be trans-
cutaneous nerve stimulation (TENS), biomagnetics and
electrotherapy.

This third category causes Becker a great deal of concern because
of the biological hazards implicit in electrical and magnetic
fields, the very subject of his book. He is almost a lone voice in
pointing out the potential dangers of nuclear magnetic resonance
imaging (MRI scans), so much the medical craze today. This
investigative process subjects the body to huge magnetic fields
and, as Becker explains, is probably not without theoretical risk,
though this has never been properly addressed as an issue.

In the late 1960s Becker was probably the first person to predict that the magnetic field of the brain extends outside the head. He remembers how his idea was ridiculed by the audience at a scientific meeting of the time. Yet, he was eventually proved correct. This leads naturally to SQUIDs (without tentacles!)...

THANK YOU, MR JOSEPHSON

Finally today, we have gone on to develop instruments for the detection of biological energy fields. Notable among these is a device called the SQUID magnetometer. SQUID is an acronym for super-conducting quantum interference device. It is opening up a whole new world of bio-energetic science. The life field can be seen and mapped with an accuracy and sensitivity that would have been unthinkable 30 years ago.

The SQUID is based on a phenomenon known as the Josephson effect, after Brian Josephson, who predicted it in 1962 while working as a graduate student at the University of Cambridge (Massachusetts). He received the 1973 Nobel Prize for his work. What his hypothesis means is that electrons, although we consider them particles (matter), can pass right through insulators as if they were waves. Such a thing is impossible in the classical physics world, but natural enough in the quantum domain. We call this tunnelling and we now know that Nature has many examples of this, including events inside the human body!

A SQUID consists of a Josephson detector, with an array of input coils to capture the bio-magnetic field, plus the necessary electronics to amplify and make sense out of the signal thus received. The whole set-up is immersed in liquid helium which makes the device exceedingly sensitive to magnetic fields, such as the delicate ones given off by living tissues and organs.

MEASURING LIFE

What can we do with such a sensitive device? One of the first biological experiments with a SQUID was carried out by John Zimmerman, who developed the SQUID, and his colleague David Cohen at MIT's National Magnet Laboratory in Cambridge, Massachusetts, in 1970. They showed the heart's magnetic field with vivid clarity. In fact, it was still detectable 15 feet from the body.

Around the turn of the century, Dutch physician Willem Einthoven discovered electrical discharges from the heart. He received the Nobel Prize for Medicine in 1924 for this work. Nowadays routine electrocardiography is a standard part of the medical technological armoury.

Each heart beat is the result of an electrical discharge within the heart muscle; the current spreads to nearby tissues and can even be detected in the feet and hands. It travels in the blood which, being a salt solution, is an excellent conductor.

In 1821 Hans Christian Oersted showed that whenever an electric current flows in a conductor, a magnetic field is formed. If the current varies (flux) then the magnetism is even more intense. But the heart's magnetic field is very weak in ordinary terms, since the current is low. However, in 1963 Gerhard Baule and Richard McFee at the Electrical Engineering Department of Syracuse University, New York, used a pair of two million-turn coils (coils with one million loops of wire – that is, wrapped around the spindle one million times) on the chest of a subject and for the first time detected the heart's field.

It was in the same year that the tunnelling or Josephson effect was first published. Now SQUIDs can map the body's heart and other biological magnetic fields with amazing sensitivity. In 1971 Cohen went on to develop a brain magneto-gram or MEG (magneto-encephalogram). The brain's field proved to be hundreds of times weaker than the heart field, necessitating that the patient be electromagnetically shielded in the room where readings take place. Clothing must be free of any magnetic material, such as zippers, snaps and nails in shoes.

Since then there has been a real explosion in monitoring biological magnetic energy fields. It turns out that biomagnetic fields are often more indicative of events taking place within the body than are electrical measurements taken at the skin surface. For example, the eye acts as a remarkable battery and produces a substantial field which increases with the amount of light falling on the retina; we can obtain and study retinograms. Cohen himself, in 1980, reported detection of steady magnetic activity from growing hair follicles! Every muscle action creates a field effect outside the body. SQUIDs even show that there is more intense cortical activity in finger control areas of the brains of musicians than non-performers.[10]

All this adds up to the fact that our living organisms are a field of teeming magnetic energy. There are other fields, too. These reflect what is going on within the body and, of course, it is entirely possible to influence the body in return. We live outside our skins! Life itself is an energy phenomenon. It no longer makes sense to practise medicine based on a biochemical or material paradigm; it's time to move over to the energy model.

So we can see that the magical, the mystical, the trendy and what was once dismissed as hocus-pocus in fact has a very sound theoretical basis in physics and can now be measured objectively, using the necessary scientific instruments.

RUPERT SHELDRAKE

We can conclude our list of thinkers by looking at the subject of information in biology. The view has long been held that all information needs some structural matter or energy system on which to be imprinted, otherwise it would have no existence in reality. It is now felt that information is somehow deeper than even energy systems; that information underpins physical reality and, especially, biological life systems. If this is the case, then energy is taking its orders from information fields.

In his book *A New Science of Life*, zoologist Rupert Sheldrake argues that all systems are regulated by something more than just matter and energy.[11] He hypothesizes that there are invisible organizing fields he calls morphogenic fields (morpho = form, genesis = making or giving birth to). These are informational fields, because they contain the detail needed to create the form, but they are not energy and therefore at this moment we cannot see them or make contact. We don't know how.

Since energy is not involved, neither are time and space. It follows therefore that the field does not attenuate with distance, as is the case with all forms of energy. It would also follow from these properties that fields can propagate effects across space and time in any direction, meaning past, present and future, here, there and everywhere at once. Actually, what Sheldrake is doing here is dressing up what we used to call 'magic' or 'supernatural' in the verbal metaphors of our age. It sounds plausible and therefore gets round resistance from die-hard thinkers. He can't prove his hypothesis, but it is attractive and self-sufficient; it covers many phenomena with no previous explanation. This theory has my vote.

According to Sheldrake's hypothesis, whenever one member of a species learns new behaviour, the causative field for the whole species changes. This would explain the famous '100 Monkeys' effect. It also suggests that the dawning of the Age of Aquarius is more likely to be real than metaphor; that human consciousness is indeed going through some kind of collective evolutionary transformation.

Sheldrake's vision is hot stuff. He's a real scientific subversive, because it throws out Darwinian evolution and turns biology on its head. You can imagine the resistance to his theories based on the old scientific principle: *it can't be true, therefore it isn't*. If we had stuck to that one we would never have had vaccination, rockets, TV, anaesthetics, motorcars or heavier-than-air flight.

The fact is that thinkers ever since Darwin have been struck by the two snags in the plausibility of his theories:

1 There isn't enough time for the progress we see, supposing only the probability of Darwinian-style evolution.
2 There is nothing to say that new species were not created by some higher conscious control, even if 'natural selection' would subsequently favour their advancement. In other words, consciousness, implicate order or some other non-material force could be running the whole show and what we observe would be just the same. In short, Darwin's theory doesn't exactly fit the facts, but the idea of a creative, intelligent cosmos with a guiding force that favours the life process over and above the mechanics of Newtonian physics certainly does.

We have made contact with Eastern philosophy!

CHAPTER 3

BIOLOGY BEYOND THE SKIN

One thing which the scientific scrutiny of biological energy is enabling us to do is re-evaluate older Oriental and other models of health, vitalism and body energetic properties. Often we find surprising concordance, and the realization is gradually dawning in the West that other models are not arcane or naïve constructs born out of ignorance but simply strange words attached to a very precise and more or less demonstrable and accurate body of knowledge.

This chapter proposes to visit some of these other models, the Chinese and Indian in particular. Each has aspects of which we will certainly need on our journey into Virtual Medicine.

THE CHINESE MODEL

Chinese philosophy, upon which Traditional Chinese Medicine (TCM) is naturally based, recognized an underlying ultimate reality which unifies everything. It was known as *Tao*, but this should not be confused with the later use of the same term by Confucius and his followers, meaning 'a path in life' or a code of conduct. In its original sense Tao means something very like our quantum field or zero-point energy; it is seen as something uniquely dynamic in character, flowing, ever-changing, creative and continuous. Thus the whole basis of TCM is energy and information; it is definitely *not* a substance-based medical model.

Tao also has the quality of being somewhat reflexive and circular – that is, coming back on itself, repeating endlessly rather than being linear. 'Returning is the motion of the Tao,' says the great classic *Tao Te Ching* by Lao Tzu, which also says 'Going far means returning'. This too reminds us of the new physics, which is teaching us a new reality that is flexible, flowing, reflexive and certainly non-linear. Effects become their own causes.

The well-known symbol the Tai-Ch'i T'u shows these several elements: change, movement, dark and light, circular, returning and complementary balance.

The two dots symbolize the fact that when one reaches the outer limit of a certain trend it must then reverse and come back on itself; each form or event contains the seeds of its own opposite. That's an awful lot of philosophy in one small motif!

Ancient Chinese medical theory is really a whole *gestalt* (composite) and it is somewhat artificial to separate out the parts. Life energy is called *Ch'i* and it flows in and around the body, constantly changing, interacting and influencing the physical domain. Blockages and disruption of the free flow of Ch'i is seen as the basis of disease. Other aspects of TCM include balance of energies (yin and yang), the five key elements (earth, air, water, wood and metal), the body clock (different organs dominant at different hours of the day) and the concept of Earth energies, or Feng Shui, interacting with all in a harmonious totality.

But what we are most concerned with here is acupuncture, the medical art of unblocking and balancing the flow of Ch'i energy through the *meridians*, or invisible energy channels, which run through and around the body. The practice of acupuncture goes back over 4,000 years, but its great flowering was the publication of a book called *Huang Ti Nei Ching* around 400 BC (*The Yellow Emperor's Classic of Internal Medicine*) available in translation by Ilza Veith [Berkeley, CA: University of California Press, 1993]. The use of fine metal needles, inserted at key points in the body in order to stimulate Ch'i, was evidently first introduced about this time also.

WHAT IS CH'I?

Ch'i is the word used to denote the vital breath or energy which pervades and animates all the cosmos. This sounds similar to the quantum information field or vacuum in which virtual particles come and go. Understanding the manifestation of Ch'i is central to TCM. It is also a key concept in which our Virtual Medicine theories come into direct contact with ancient wisdom, since there are remarkable parallels between descriptions of quantum probability fields and texts about Ch'i.

> When the Ch'i condenses, its visibility becomes apparent so that these are then seen as shapes (of individual things). When it disperses, its visibility is no longer apparent and there are no shapes. At the time of its condensation, can one say otherwise than this is temporary? But at its time of dispersing, can one hastily say that it is then non-existent?[1]

This brilliant insight is quite remarkable. How could the author of this ancient text know that in centuries to come quantum physics would show that indeed the cosmos, far from being a vacuum containing fixed matter, would be seen instead as pervaded with information fields which cause 'matter' (virtual particles) to come and go as they need when interacting with something else? Again, our understanding of the true nature of disease turns on this point: if information energy of a disease is present but the disease not apparent, is it truly manifest? Or do we have to wait until structure alters and decays before we allow ourselves to be interested in healing? It is a crucial question, since now for the first time with Virtual Medicine we are able to see the forward projection of disease, *before* it becomes apparent.

In the human body Ch'i flows through discreet pathways called meridians and these affect the vitality and function of the organs. A blockage in a meridian will result in a malfunction of any organ through which it passes. It is worth pointing out here that a meridian passes through more than one organ and a disturbance in the meridian need not be confined to that organ alone. Thus for example the gallbladder meridian transects the canine tooth (eye tooth), upper and lower, as it passes across the face. An abscess in these teeth can cause gall-bladder dysfunction and vice versa.

Not only that, but we can bring in the 'organ clock' notion described in the *Nei Ching*. The gall-bladder meridian is dominant between 11 p.m. and 1 a.m. Thus the toothache is likely to be at its worst around midnight. Observations of this sort often astonish patients but are simple when you have the right medical model.

The Winds of Change

The meridians have been a source of great fascination to doctors and laymen alike in the West. Because of the craving for anatomical certainty, there has been a continued search to find some kind of structural explanation for the existence of meridians. They are clearly not nerve channels, blood vessels or any kind of duct system. Since no obvious anatomical structures mimic the described pathways of meridians, the tendency for Western science has been to dismiss the concept as something fanciful; this has not been helped by the choice of unusual metaphorical names given certain points such as *The Sea of Energy* (Conception Vessel 6), *The Marshes of the Wind* (Bladder 12) and *The Door of the Mental* (Heart 7).

Gradually the climate has changed. During the 1960s and 1970s the world's attention was increasingly drawn to Chinese traditions, partly accelerated by President Nixon's visit to mainland China. At around that time we first saw dramatic TV footage of major operations being carried out with no more anaesthetic than needles placed at exactly the right places in the skin. It was obvious to all and sundry that acupuncture worked, and worked at least as well as Western scientific medicine in some surprising ways, no matter how alien the rhetoric and however unfamiliar the mechanics and model. Since then, science has begun probing to see if it can establish at least some objective evidence for the Chinese model (evidence, that is, within its own paradigm and criteria of judgement).

We seem to have made a certain amount of progress.

THE NATURE OF MERIDIANS

In February 1937 the prestigious *British Medical Journal* carried an article by Sir Thomas Lewis describing a hitherto unknown network of cutaneous nerves.[2] He called it the 'nocifensor system' and deduced, from his experiments, that it was an independent cutaneous nerve system, unrelated to known pathways and unconnected to the autonomic nervous system. It was composed, not of nerve fibres, but a network of thin lines, similar to meridians.

In 1985 Pierre de Vernejoul at the University of Paris carried out a definitive and much-quoted experiment. He used a radioactive marker, technetium 99m, which he injected into subjects at classic acupuncture points. He then used gamma-camera imaging to track the subsequent movement of the isotope. He was able to show that the tracer migrated along the classic meridian lines, travelling quite quickly: a distance of 30 cm in 4–6 minutes.[3] As a control he made a number of random injections into the skin (*not* at acupuncture points) and also injected the tracer directly into veins and lymphatic channels. There was no significant migration of the tracer at other sites than an acupuncture point. What this simple but helpful study proved beyond doubt is that meridians are definitely real 'vessels' but they conform to no macroscopic anatomical structures whatever.

So if meridians are not nerve-conducting channels or other anatomically visible vessels, what are they? How is the energy conducted?

The answer is almost certainly via the collagen fibres of the connective tissues. As the name suggests, connective tissue fills in between the main organs and layers. There is thus a continuum of liquid crystalline water-bound collagen fibres running throughout the whole body. Recent studies have shown that these are not just mechanical fibres but that they have dielectric and conductive properties which make them sensitive to pressure, pH, local ionic composition and surrounding electromagnetic fields. In fact these collagen fibres, like a network mesh of fine electrical fibrils, form the ideal conductor medium in which many of the electro-magnetic phenomena described in this book may take place.

Even just disturbing and stressing these fibres gives off an electrical potential. You will notice when you have electro-acupuncture, as described in the Chapter 4, that the practitioner has the knack of 'massaging' the point he or she is testing, to wake it up and release this electrical potential in order to make a successful reading.

Remarkably, and very conveniently for us, this network of semi-conductor material can enforce a one-direction flow on the electrical current, acting rather like an electrical circuit with one-way gates called diodes. Once again, scientific testing has validated ancient wisdom and shown that the acupuncture meridians flow in one direction only – that which was described by the original *Nei Ching* text.

Body Consciousness

The collagen network is of course in contact with the intracellular chemical fluid medium; this matrix in total provides an excitable continuum for rapid, coherent intercommunication throughout the whole living system of a human body. It is further the origin of the DC body field, as described by Saxton Burr and later Robert Becker (see Chapter 2).

This previously unknown dielectric domain could be described as a kind of body consciousness, separate from the brain and nerve cells, which is able to detect and retain experiences as a kind of memory, as well as register new experiences.

Interestingly, the fact that bound water plays an important role in consciousness was shown by evidence that anaesthesia may act by displacing bound water from membrane interfaces. Becker reported that general anaesthesia leads to a complete attenuation of the DC body field.[4] I have already remarked that acupuncture can render the conscious patient anaesthetized. Add this to the knowledge that some surgical patients feel pain even when (ostensibly) unconscious, and we can readily admit that brain and body consciousness are not the same and can be decoupled one from the other.

THE AYURVEDIC MODEL

The ancient Ayurvedic healing tradition is considerably older than TCM, indeed is probably the oldest surviving model of health and disease. It has certainly stood the test of time and therefore deserves to be accorded respect. It would also prompt the wise scientist to begin asking what is workable about a system which has endured so long.

Once again, the zero-ground information field concept comes in: this time it is called *Brahman*, the ultimate reality. It is the soul or inner essence of everything and far transcends the ability to describe it in words (remember the difficulties of describing anything quite as weird as quantum physics). The word *maya* is used to describe how the ultimate reality of everything is made manifest in perceivable forms. It is often said that maya means the world is an illusion. Well, thanks to quantum mechanics we know this to be true at the subatomic level!

The universal energy, which the Chinese call Ch'i, is here known as *prana*. Instead of the meridians, the Indian system introduces the concept of *chakras*. These are the gates or channels by which the life-giving universal prana energy enters (and leaves) our bodies, thus influencing our bodily functions and vitality.

There are seven main chakras. Each one of these has a correspondence with anatomical structures, notably a nerve plexus and an endocrine gland. The name and correspondence of these main chakras is:

CHAKRA	NERVE PLEXUS	ENDOCRINE GLAND
Base	sacro-coccygeal	*gonads*
Sacral	sacral	*Leydig cells in gonads*
Solar plexus	solar plexus	*adrenals*
Heart	heart plexus	*thymus*
Throat	cervical ganglia	*thyroid*
Head	hypothalamus/pituitary	*pituitary*
Crown	cerebral cortex	*pineal*

What is less widely known is that texts refer also to other energy centres associated with major joint structures of the body, like the knees, ankles, elbows, etc. Taken altogether there are over 360 chakras of the body. These in turn are said to be joined together by a network of etheric channels called *nadis*, which are interwoven with the nervous system. Thus, unlike the TCM meridian system, chakras and nadis display considerable correspondence with anatomical structures.

Can we say anything about the chakras? What we need is hard evidence of their existence and significance. Unfortunately, this is singularly lacking. The best work to date seems to be that of Japanese psychic and clinical psychologist Hiroshi Motoyama. He is also a high priest and a yogi adept of some ability. At his research faculty, the Institute for Religious Psychology, he developed the AMI scanner, an acronym for Apparatus for Measuring the Functional Conditions of Meridians and their Corresponding Internal Organs (see Chapter 4).

Motoyama also claimed he had developed a 'Chakra Instrument' able to detect minute electrical, magnetic and optical variables in the immediate environment shell of the study subject.[5] The detectors have to be used in a light-proof room, shielded by lead sheeting on the walls and lined with foil which is

Chakra points

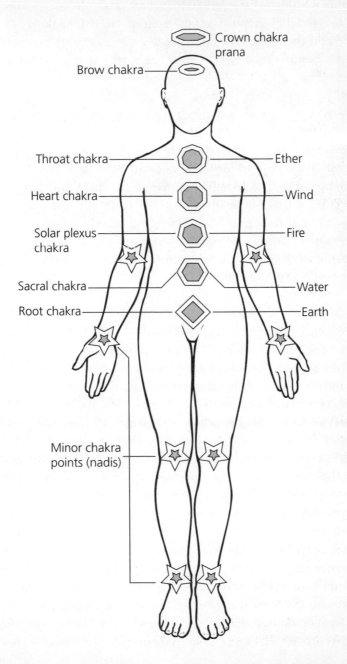

Crown chakra
prana

Brow chakra

Throat chakra — Ether

Heart chakra — Wind

Solar plexus chakra — Fire

Sacral chakra — Water

Root chakra — Earth

Minor chakra points (nadis)

grounded, to keep the electrical potential at zero. A 10-cm copper disc plus a photovoltaic cell (which generates electricity when light is detected) is positioned in front of the chakra being 'sensed', off the body. The magnetic detector is simply placed on the floor beside the subject – in other words within his or her magnetic field.

Changes in readings are processed and stored by a multichannel recorder, along with a number of conventional variables such as respiration rate, ECG and galvanic skin response (similar to a lie detector). Using questionnaires and evaluating disease susceptibility and organ function, and intercalating that with his 'detector' readings, Motoyama claims to have had some degree of success in objectifying the chakras. However the obvious criticism seems to be that he is depending heavily on the correlation between chakras and nerve plexuses. He could arguably be measuring nothing more than autonomic nerve activity, not energy vortexes in the ether!

SPIN

On the subject of vortices, this is probably a good opportunity to describe the phenomenon that practitioners using the systems described later in the book call 'spin'. In physics there is a phenomenon known as 'optical rotation', which comes from the helical structure of crystalline solids, or helical molecules in liquids and solutions. Spin is designated either right or left (dextro- or laevo-).

What practitioners with Virtual Medicine detector equipment have come up with is that healthy blood and saliva have a right-spin; urine and faeces have left-spin. When a person is under considerable duress or experiencing geopathic stress, this reverses.

Is it relevant? Certainly. Many patients with 'reverse spin' will not recover therapeutically until the spin is back to normal. The truth may be that spin-reversal makes one susceptible to outside events, such as geopathic stress, rather than vice versa.

But spin could have far wider implications. In 1995 I attended a conference in St Petersburg, in common with many other colleagues from the Scientific and Medical Network (a group of doctors and scientists dedicated to finding out more about the metaphysical and transcendent aspects of creation). There we heard lecture after lecture from leading Russian scientists about the properties of what are known as *torsion fields*.

Matter, we now know, has three basic physical properties: charge, mass and spin. Each of these gives rise to a characteristic field. Charge creates an electromagnetic field, mass gives rise to a gravitational field, and spin generates what we call a torsion field. It was high-level stuff, but what we learned is that torsion fields are different in having instantaneous effects at all points. Gravity fields have a distance effect, and electro-magnetic propagation has a time (frequency) effect, even though the ruling speed of light is pretty fast! Torsion fields, almost by definition, have neither a distance nor a time effect. In other words, we were hearing about a model which could explain telepathy and other supposedly etheric phenomena, which are so often dismissed as totally implausible.

I repeat once again my often-stated woe that if only doctors (and many other scientists) knew enough current physics, so much that seems strange and therefore improbable would yield to common sense enquiry. I was particularly pleased at the St Petersburg conference to hear through our discussions that thought could almost certainly be imprinted in space outside our skulls and left there for others to 'walk into'. There was a perfectly scientific explanation for certain strange and creepy feelings many of us experience from time to time. It could be the basis of déjà vu, though my Tunnels of Time project means I am heavily committed to the validity of past lives.

The potential for health effects from torsion fields, especially some of the strange outer-limit manifestations that you will read about in this text, is of course considerable. Readers will be able to work out many ways in which this obscure but enriching model could apply to the body-mind-spirit composite we call our Being.

WHAT ABOUT AURAS?

There is evident confusion about what is meant by an aura. Some consider it to be simply the energy shell around a person, which can become visible in certain circumstances. Others think it has metaphysical import. People claim to be able to see many layers of aura, which they attribute to the mental, emotional, astral and other aspects of the individual's composite being. I can only say that few can do this and therefore it is not truly objective. Further confusion is added by the fact that even I can see 'auras' around buildings, rocks and other formations, if the lighting and climatic conditions are right.

With this in mind, what objective evidence is there for such a thing as an aura? We will assume that it is identical with the L-Field or bio-plasma body mentioned in Chapter 2. There have been various attempts to make the total aura of a person visible. In 1911 Dr Walter Kilner, working at a London hospital, published a book entitled *The Human Atmosphere or the Aura Made Visible with the Aid of Chemical Screens*. He invented the Kilner screen, which was effectively a pair of glasses in which double screens held a liquid containing dicyanogen blue dissolved in alcohol.

Kilner described three zones around the body:

1 a thin dark layer close to the skin
2 a more vaporous layer, with rays pointing away from the skin
3 a tenuous outer layer about 6 inches across, with varying density and colours.

He found that this 'aura' would change with age, sex, mental energy and health factors. He was able to see shadows in the aura and could tentatively diagnose diseases such as hepatitis, cancer, appendicitis, epilepsy and psychological states.

Nowadays we can buy 'aura glasses' on the Internet. These are glasses with specially coated lenses which allow through only certain colours and screen out incident light. Some practice and concentration is required, but by all accounts most people can master it.

But the most definitive work to date in this field is the often-quoted study carried out by Dr Valerie Hunt and others at UCLA in 1977.[6] She had already discovered, using electromyography (EMG), that the body emits hitherto undetected oscillations between the 'noise' of normal muscle contractions. Using these as a marker she was studying the aura-energetic effects of a soft-tissue-manipulation healing technique called Rolfing (after Dr Ida P. Rolf, who 50 years ago called her work *structural integration*). To do this Hunt wired the subject to EMG electrodes positioned at the site of each major chakra, relayed to a recording booth where the sophisticated equipment monitored fluctuations in the electro-magnetic energy of the body.

But how to visualize the aura? Hunt brought in a trained psychic observer, Rosalyn Bruyere, who apparently could see human auras and the changes which took place in them. But was this really true? Hunt arranged to have Bruyere's descriptions and comments recorded synchronously with the changes in electro-magnetic measurements.

While the Rolfing therapy was taking place, Bruyere, who was obviously not allowed to see the physical recordings at this stage, reported changes in the colour and form of the energetic fields of the patient and Rolfer. Most satisfyingly, the patient and healer auras merged towards the end of the session as one identical shape and colour, something often described subjectively by hands-on energy healers and their patients.

The real test came when the recordings and aura descriptions were de-coded. It was found that changes in the patient's EMG status corresponded exactly with altered descriptions from Bruyere. Not only that, but when the frequency figures were subjected to mathematical analysis the Hertz bands suggested colours which also exactly corresponded with Bruyere's descriptions.

It is not too much to propose from this study that many energy healers get their results by superimposing a strong and reasonably balanced auric field (their own) onto the patient's disturbed and sick field; a version of shunomatism mentioned in Chapter 2. This isn't such an infringement as it sounds, since the two beings work together and seem to 'evolve' a new energetic unity that is somewhat bigger and beyond either one of them. This higher unity is able to heal and nurture.

MEASURING CHIGUNG

Most people today have heard of Tai Ch'i and its remarkable health benefits. Chigung is a more disciplined meditation, also using the power of Ch'i. Like acupuncture, this ancient practice is based on meridian theory. It is usually done sitting still with 'regulation' of breath (a relaxed concentration). Practitioners learn to monitor consciously the flow of Ch'i through meridians and channels in their bodies. Advanced practitioners can emit Ch'i with sufficient intensity that it can help others' ailing energies, forming the basis of yet another kind of energetic healing. There is also, evidently, an inhibiting Ch'i.

This ought to be detectable by scientific instruments. I have observed the beneficial effects on electro-dermal screening test methods discussed later in this book. But a more academic study was carried out by a group in the US and published in the *American Journal of Chinese Medicine* in 1991. Using infrared detectors, the researchers were able to measure output from the palms of advanced Chigung practitioners and concluded that at least part of the emitted Ch'i was in the infrared band of the electromagnetic spectrum. They were also able to show measurable levels of enhancing Ch'i emissions on human fibroblasts and boar (porcine) sperm. Facilitating Ch'i increased DNA synthesis, protein synthesis and cell growth in the human cells, while inhibiting Ch'i decreased all three. In the case of the boar sperm, different tests established that facilitating Ch'i increased respiration 12–13 per cent, while inhibiting Ch'i decreased it some 45–48 per cent.[7]

There no longer need be any doubt that science has crossed over into what was considered the etheric and is able to show a real effect. Of course measurements are made of electro-magnetic changes, not at the quantum level. But the body itself acts as the most sensitive quantum detector we have. Whatever is happening out there, it is real, not magic.

Now, surprisingly, we have machines which are actually capable of *generating Ch'i*. This is remarkable, because Ch'i masters have always felt that only living things could generate Ch'i. Even today, the only real detector of Ch'i is a sensitive and aware human being (a bio-detector). Dr Yuri Khronos, working with an Eastern-trained Ch'i master named Dong Chen, has been able to produce Ch'i electronically. Not only that, but it can be broadcast from tapes played through normal hi-fi loudspeaker units. Ch'i-aware people report rapid changes in their states of awareness from such broadcast recordings.

It is only a matter of time before Ch'i detectors are made. The impact of this on the development of consciousness is hard to foresee but will certainly be important (see Chapter 14).

PHOTOGRAPHS CANNOT LIE: OR CAN THEY?

In 1939 Semyon D. Kirlian, a Russian technician, was repairing hospital equipment when he noticed something strange. It was another case of the right mind prepared to benefit from a chance event; Kirlian thought it through properly and went on, with his wife, to develop what we now call Kirlian photography.

What he had discovered was that by the interaction of a very high-frequency electric discharge and a photographic plate, energy imprints of living organisms can be revealed on the film. The subject, enclosed in a light-tight bag, is in contact with a charged metal plate backed onto a photographic emulsion. At the moment of discharge, high-energy electrons jump from the plate to the subject, resulting in ionization of a thin layer of air between the two. The photographic emulsion is excited in the normal way and can be developed to reveal what may best be described as a visualization of the subject's energy field (which may or may not be the same as the aura).

Further research by scientists at the Kirov State University of Kazakhstan extended the discovery. They found that the light emanated was polarized (blue or red-yellow). This seems to accord with the traditional Chinese view of yin and yang energies.[8] These scientists began to refer to the visible energy shell beyond the body surface that was being recorded as *the bioplasmic body*. Studies showed it was affected by atmospheric conditions and cosmic events, such as sunspots. The Kirlians had already noticed rapid and pronounced changes in the energy photographed, caused by emotional disturbance. Increased light seemed to pour out with anger and (perhaps surprisingly) exhaustion. So here we seem to be looking at an actual visual confirmation of Burr's L-Fields.

Experiments with plants and animals showed that each had a unique, defining energy field. What is most impressive is that even if half a leaf is cut away, the Kirlian photograph still shows the full field, the whole leaf energy appearing to be present even when the cut-away particles or mass is absent. Could it also be that the leaf 'ghost' photograph is defining one of Sheldrake's morphogenic fields? If not, what holds the energy vibration in place? It must surely be an information field of some kind.

The Kazakhstan workers also tried to record objectively the bio-physical changes that may take place in the hands of healers when treating a patient. What was visualized on the print when the hands of the healer were held close to a patient under the Kirlian camera was a narrow stream of energy, concentrating into an intense band which streamed into the area of the illness. What appeared to be happening was the transfer of energy from the bio-plasmic body of the healer to that of the patient.[9]

Other applications of the photography, to demonstrate energetic transference of vital energy to water or seeds which had been held in the hands of a talented healer, were also successful. Photographs of manufactured or junk food show that it lacks the vital energy field which is present in and around fresh or whole food. The conclusion seems too obvious to comment upon.

In 1953 Dr M. K. Gaikin, a Leningrad surgeon, made an interesting discovery. He realized that the position of the main flares on the skin, which are characteristic of Kirlian photographs of humans, did not correspond to anything anatomical – but that they did appear at classical acupuncture points!

Naturally there has been hope that Kirlian photography will be able to offer the means to diagnose disease, based on imaging changes in the bioplasmic body. However, to date there seems considerable difficulty in distinguishing artefacts from true or meaningful photographic phenomena. Perhaps this may change in time. But for the present, few except the dedicated core of enthusiasts seem to take this remarkable technique very seriously. Thus Kirlian photography still has mainly the status of a party trick or an engaging exhibit at psychic fairs and carnivals, where practitioners charge a small fee for a 'picture of your aura'. Ironically, most of these aura-simulation cameras are not true Kirlians. There has to be direct contact with the plate, impossible at even a tiny distance or through a lens.

NOGIER'S SYSTEM

I conclude this brief survey of biology outside of our skin by introducing an odd offshoot of acupuncture theory called ear or auriculo-acupuncture. It was somewhat of a lost art but has been re-developed, particularly by French neurosurgeon Dr Paul Nogier. His system is based upon the image of a foetus projected onto the external ear and includes some 200 points. It has become widely adopted, even in China, where it has sparked a wave of research into the apparent embryonic connections.

Historically the Chinese, Arabs, Romanies, Hindus and some Europeans advocated needling a point on the ear lobe to remedy eye deficiencies. Even today some European doctors recommend the insertion of a gold or silver earring to stimulate this spot continuously in cases of eye deficiency. Currently auriculo-acupuncture is much used for anaesthesia, obesity and addictions such as smoking. An ancient Indian text, the *Suchi Veda* (which translated means 'Science of Needle Piercing') gives detailed techniques and points for needling the ears. It is interesting that the Arabs should use the ear mainly for the treatment of low back pain and kidney trouble, when it is known that the ear is seen by the Chinese as the outward 'flowering' of the kidneys.[10]

The purpose is not to discuss the method here but to offset it somewhat against what was discussed earlier about the proving of meridians. If Nogier's theory is correct and there are connections from the ear points to each individual organ, we find

ourselves very unsettled on the idea that meridians are anatomically proven. Indeed, it rather opens the debate up again. What had Nogier discovered? There is no arguing his powers of observation; many other people have confirmed the efficacy and accuracy of his correlations. But it does not rely on the concept of independent energy channels running through the body.

Rather, I think, Nogier's idea is one of neurological energy conduits projecting into the body field, and perhaps we come back to Sir Thomas Lewis' idea of the nocifensor system, though this is entirely personal view of mine. What encourages me to make this speculation is, firstly, that it clearly is not meridian-based and, secondly, a consideration of the method of allergy testing taught me years ago and known as the auriculo-cardiac reflex or ACR. I describe it briefly in two of my former books.[11] The great figure Avicenna used a version of this technique. A modern form of it is still taught by Dr Julian Kenyon of the Centre for the Study of Complementary Therapy in Southampton, UK.

The practitioner bases his or her diagnosis on changes in characteristics of the pulse. It is not merely that it speeds up, which is often the case, but that the point of maximum amplitude shifts away from the heart. The exact nature of the reflex in any patient is ascertained by flashing a very bright light onto any area of sympathetic nerve supply. The earlobe itself is just right for this. The resulting benchmark change of pulse is noted.

Then by bringing filters containing food and other allergy test substances over the skin of the forearm, the practitioner can recognize and grade whichever ones are hostile to the patient. Generally, the bigger the pulse disturbance, the longer it takes to settle down to normal, the more severe the allergen. What is curious about this method, and the reason for introducing it, is that *there is no necessity to touch the skin with the filters.* Simply holding the substance a centimetre or so from the surface of the body will still produce the reaction. This is a true field effect. It is based on the fact that an allergy is an information field disturbance and not merely an immunological process (see page 66).

This is a very simple virtual allergy test, without the sophisticated electronics described later.

CHAPTER 4

THE BIRTH OF ELECTRO-ACUPUNCTURE

DR REINHOLD VOLL

Enter Dr Reinhold Voll, physician extraordinary. He is the very stuff of which legends are made: dark, irascible and arrogantly conscious of his genius. Originally trained in architecture, he qualified and became interested in technology as well as preventative medicine, an ideal combination to set the stage for his future. Voll contracted cancer of the bladder but refused to accept the Western dogma of terminal decline. Instead he sought relief through the intervention of traditional acupuncture methods. Remarkably, although he needed life-long catheterization, Voll conquered the disease sufficiently to continue working for over two decades – a testimony to the effectiveness of his teachings. Many people over the years have had cause to be grateful for this minor miracle.

Voll set about the business of trying to marry up Chinese medical wisdom with Western technology, a transition which had to come sooner or later, but with Voll it came soon, and comprehensively to boot. He began to survey acupuncture points and their related meridians, using a modification of a standard valve ohmmeter which he called the *diatherapuncteur*, and with it he founded the science of 'electro-acupuncture' in the 1950s. You may also at times hear of the *dermatron*, a later transistorized version of the same instrument.

The patient holds one electrode while the investigating physician uses a probe to complete the circuit by touching the skin at the point being tested. The small tip of the probe allows remarkable accuracy of placement, yet yields a great deal of information other than just skin resistance, as we shall see. The current is in the region of 10 – 12 microamps at a potential of 1.0 – 1.25 volts.

In other words, quite safe. Any more and the current itself would become stimulating and produce changes, instead of monitoring status quo. Indeed, just the very act of pressing firmly on the acupuncture point is sufficient to stimulate it, and very sensitive patients may even feel unwell due to this effect after such a test session.

Voll's first interesting discovery was that almost all Chinese acupuncture points are detectable by a change in skin resistance at that spot and are remarkably accurately located; most are within a millimetre or two of where the classic texts say. At these sites the skin resistance is a fairly constant 95,000 ohms (elsewhere the skin is highly insulating, at around 2 million ohms, except when wet). However, Voll also found many more such points than the *Nei Ching* and other classic texts tell us. So far this is simply a matter of scientific detection and there can be no argument; anyone who wants to measure these points for themselves can do so easily.

Additional Vessels

There are 12 main acupuncture meridians recognized in TCM and two principle governor vessels running in the midline, front and back (Conception Vessel and Governor Meridian, respectively).

It very quickly became obvious to Voll that there were other conducting channels, many extra points, and at least eight new 'vessels' were mapped, then labelled according to what he felt they represented in terms of biological function, namely: *lymphatic drainage, nervous system* (including the autonomic nervous system), *fatty degeneration* (including fat-soluble toxic chemical deposits), *organ decay* (including malignancy), *nonmalignant cystic fibrous and other benign degenerations, skin, joints* and *allergies*. His system brought the total up to 20 bi-lateral channels, two to each digit, fingers and toes, making a total of 40 channels in all.

There has also been the opportunity to rename some of the classic meridians with names more in line with modern Western science; thus the Chinese 'triple-warmer' has become linked with the endocrine system; the circulation-sex meridian (heart master) is now linked with vascular degeneration.

The illustration below shows the hands and feet and each vessel named on the Voll system. The only asymmetry is that the channel on the medial side of each big toe differs; on the left foot it is taken as indicative of *spleen* function, whereas on the right foot the same vessel is named for the *pancreas*.

Hand

Foot

Too Much or Too Little Energy Flowing?

From here on it starts to become increasingly contentious. What Voll did is to arrange that a normal 'balanced' reading on a true acupuncture point is set at 50. At the upper end, 100, this would represent no resistance to current flow. A reading of 0 would mean total resistance (no current flowing whatever). Readings significantly higher than 50 on this scale mean too much energy (this may not at first sound an obvious problem, but remember all such excess energy must be stolen from somewhere else).

Generally we take readings of 65 or more to mean an excitation (or irritation). Over 80 is an active inflammatory process and over 90 an active inflammatory process that is pronounced in grade.

Conversely, readings below 50 mean degeneration and decay, which is more serious because destructive changes are less readily reversed. Below 40 is considered a sign of danger and below 30 an indication of an already established cancer or dead tissue (for example, I have observed readings as low as 27 at the point representing the defunct adrenal gland of a case of Addison's disease but without malignancy being present). I know of no EAV practitioner who has recorded less than 20 on this scale of values, but it would represent the final stages of tissue degeneration and death.

The scale of pathological readings is shown here schematically:

Value	Significance
90–100	Total '-itis'. Whole organ inflamed
80–89	Partial '-itis'
70–79	Cumulative irritations, premorbid
60–69	Physiological irritant values only
48–59	Normal range of variability
40–47	Incipient degeneration
30–39	Serious degeneration, pre-malignant
20–29	Advanced degeneration, almost certain malignancy
Under 20	Degeneration in the final stages

This may summed up as: *increasingly serious inflammatory and active organ disease above 80; serious degeneration and risk of malignancy below 40.*

Indicator Drop

In addition to the general level of readings, Voll recognized another phenomenon, which is where the reading is fine at first but after a few seconds it begins to die away to a lower level. What was *observed* is that the meridian somehow could not hold on to its energy. The *interpretation* of this is that there is disease tissue present somewhere in the indicated tissue of that meridian, influencing the energy levels.

Voll called this phenomenon the Indicator Drop (ID), and he considered this to be the most important reading of all. It points clearly to some significant pathological process taking place, regardless of what level the initial reading was found to measure. Put another way, a meridian which is high but where there is no Indicator Drop is not nearly so much a problem as one which reads nearer 50 but has a major drop. For example, a high liver reading (90+) means a major detoxification is going on, with high liver energy and possible inflammation of liver tissue. Voll called this reading the 'speeded Indicator Drop' and declared it indicative of chemical intoxication. But providing there is no die-off effect, the problem lies elsewhere. The liver overburdening is a secondary manifestation. The source of the toxins is the matter which needs rectifying, which when solved will ease the liver problem.

Basically, the bigger the Indicator Drop, the more serious the pathology giving rise to it. The electro-acupuncture practitioner will seek out the biggest drop in the measurement system and choose to treat that first, as a priority. This leads almost inevitably to the concept of 'most stressed organ' and implies a necessary treatment regimen.

Correlations

Where Voll became decidedly controversial is the systematic way he went about trying to find correlations between each electro-acupuncture points and specific organs and diseases.

Most scholars of the Chinese system are content to view the 'gall bladder' or 'large intestine' meridians as concepts or qualities of energetic potential, rather than being related necessarily to disease of those organs. Voll thought otherwise and, over many years of painstaking and detailed research on many thousands of clinical cases, he gradually catalogued enough data to be able to associate certain points with certain organs or relevant tissues.

Gone was the old system of colourful metaphors such as *The Sea of Energy* (Conception Vessel 6) and *The Door of the Mental* (Heart 7). Instead, in Voll's system, the first point on the endocrine meridian is associated with gonadal and adrenal function; the fifth point on the heart meridian connects with the mitral valve (left) or tricuspid valve (right); the ninth point on the lung meridian is larynx, and so on (all examples counted from the tip of the relevant digit, whether the start or finish of the meridian).

Existing meridians were found to have several additional points, so a new naming system had to be devised. The first point between 1 and 2 became 1a. Then came a 1b. But then further divisions led to 1-1 and 1-2 and so on. The result is confusing but there is a certain amount of consistency based on function. For example, Voll considered the second Voll-point on each finger (just distal to the last knuckle joint) to be concerned with lymphatic drainage, so these are always designated 1-1; the point immediately proximal to the last knuckle joint he associated with the sympathetic plexus of the system concerned, and these are always designated 1a. Conveniently, Voll's method concentrates mainly on taking readings on the hands and feet and nearby skin, so the patient is spared much disrobing.

Eventually Voll published a complete knowledge system of all the above which we now call 'electro-acupuncture according to Voll', or *EAV* for short. It is the first real model of what I have chosen to call Virtual Medicine.

Criticism

As a user of the EAV method with some years' study it is possible to say that there are indeed some remarkable correlations between EAV points and meridians, but overall, I feel that Voll has invited criticism by trying to fit the clinical findings into his mental hypothesis. After doing so he has come up with a useful but partly inaccurate 'map'. That said, there is nothing that even comes close in scientific terms to such an advanced energy diagnostic system and it does indeed go a long way to combining the intuitive genius of the Chinese system with the preciseness of Western electronic technology.

Perhaps, as the idolization accorded to Voll fades into a brilliant historical perspective, it will be open to others to question some of the master's dogma and make changes which reflect more accuracy in what is being tested and more humility concerning the fallibility of the method.

Central Measurement Points (CMPs)

There are many points to measure, over a thousand in all. We don't try to measure every one on each patient. An obvious question would be: is there any way to establish quickly the general state of each meridian? One suggestion is to measure the ends of the meridians. These points are called 'Ting points' in Chinese nomenclature.

Without going into the arguments for and against, it has been settled that it is better to measure a little further up the meridian, at what we call the central measurement point or CMP. With one or two exceptions, like the thumbs, big toes and heart meridian (inside of the little finger), this point is just distal to the second knuckle joint. This gives an overall idea of the energy of that meridian. If there is suspicion of a problem then it is very simple to delve deeper and check other points related to that meridian.

By using the CMPs as quick reference points it is usually possible to home in on the problem area. However, nothing in EAV overrides the common sense of history taking. If the patient says she has lung problems and the CMP has no Indicator Drop (ID), it is mandatory to check other points on the lung meridian.

As with conventional medicine, electro-acupuncture is about establishing a hypothesis as to the causation of illness and then dealing with it. The fact that different criteria and an unfamiliar frame of reference are called into play does not alter this basic logic or mean that we ignore what clues there may be in the patient's description of his or her problem.

PRACTICAL CONSIDERATIONS OF EAV

EAV is not easy, though simple enough in concept. It is rumoured that it takes five years to make a good EAV specialist. That may be true, but being able to get useful readings and helpful therapy pointers can be learned in a matter of days. After all, one does not need to be a brain surgeon to learn to dress wounds and set up an intravenous line. Consistency of probe pressure is the hard part to master. Once the practitioner can do that, everything else follows.

The real difficulty is to learn the remedies. It's a whole different repertory (see Chapter 7) and certainly does take years to get to grips with. But there are always textbooks to help.

It is also important to respect certain general rules. We know, for instance, that testing after a heavy meal obscures the results. We call this a *parasympathetic dominant state*, when the patient is lethargic and the energetic system somewhat closed down (yin state). But TCM tells us more: that, as in all things, the body cycles through contrasting phases; midnight to noon is a time of sympathetic dominance (yang); noon to midnight is parasympathetic dominance (yin). Moral: don't test after about 6 p.m. and never after the patient has eaten a big meal! These are things one learns gradually.

Other factors which can reduce a patient's energy are lack of sleep, severe stress, cold or medications.

Quadrant Measurement

A quick and easy test to see if the patient's energies are adequate for EAV testing is what we call *quadrant measurement*. It can be shortened to a hand-to-hand reading. Provided the energies fall in the 80–90 range, there is sufficient energy for testing. If not, some means of stimulating the patient is required. This could be having the patient run on the spot, clap his or her hands together forcefully a few times, or tap repeatedly on both temples.

Quadrant testing is a useful preliminary procedure. Readings are taken from hand-to-hand, right hand to right foot, left hand to left foot, and foot-to-foot (foot measurements are made with the patient's soles on electrode plates). If there is a significantly higher or lower reading in one of the quadrants compared to the other three, it suggests that the key pathology is in that quarter.

Hypothalamic Disorder

Sam Williams, Jr, an advanced EAV specialist physician, taught me the importance of checking hypothalamic status. It happens sometimes that when recording meridian energies at the CMPs that everything seems 'irritable' – that is, a great many small Indicator Drops register, but nothing really stands out. This makes it difficult to know where to enter the case. Systemic steroid therapy can produce a similar picture, where IDs are being clearly suppressed. However, in this case there is usually some reading which enables us to break into the problem.

Screening for hypothalamic disorder is done by measuring at the traditional Chinese point of Triple Warmer (TW) 20, which lies just above the ear pinna. Measurement is made while the patient is in contact with the ground with one hand, touching TW 20 with the probe. Alternatively, the patient uses the index finger of the hand holding the bar electrode to touch TW 20, while the therapist uses the probe on the allergy vessel CMP of the opposite side. An imbalance of readings on the two sides indicates either hypothalamus disorder, or possibly a dislocation of cervical vertebrae at the level of C3 or C4.

If one or the other condition exists, it will skew the results and it would be best to remedy this problem first. Subluxation will need a realignment manipulation by a skilled chiropractor or osteopath. If it is indeed a hypothalamus problem, matters can be improved by choosing a suitable restorative remedy or light therapy (see Chapter 9).

Unless a hypothalamus offset is corrected first, the therapy regime will not be totally accurate and consequently less effective.

Foci

Using electro-acupuncture, one is given several new insights into the disease process that are not obvious to the traditionally-orientated clinician. For example we have the concept of a 'focus' (plural: *foci*). No matter what the presentation of the patient's complaint, it often emerges that there is some area of the body which is distressed and 'transmitting' a trouble signal which influences the energy body adversely.

Common examples would be old tonsillitis, appendicitis, what I call pelvic 'anger' in a woman, prostatitis in a man or teeth and gum problems (see Chapter 12 for startling new revelations about the dangers of teeth foci). These foci can appear 'silent' clinically but they are certainly not so electromagnetically.

When a focus is active within an organ tissue it will disturb the body's homeostatic regulatory mechanism. The body needs to divert a great deal of its energies to cover up and compensate for the focal disturbance. This causes imbalances in other organs, with fatigue and global low energy states. Therapy may be blocked until the focus is corrected.

It soon becomes evident to the budding EAV specialist that these hidden and smouldering foci are quite dangerous and can create a great deal of chronic ill-health, rather like the 'smouldering virus' that we began to talk about in the 1960s. Spread of infection and toxins by blood transportation is obvious. But another largely unsuspected route is retrograde seepage along nerve channels. We know that viruses and bacteria *can* travel in nerves: rabies, herpes and poliomyelitis are just three diseases where this is known to happen. In 1923 two groups in Paris and the US chanced upon identical experiments. Each inoculated rabbits in the eye with Herpes simplex virus ('cold sore' virus) and showed clearly that the virus tracked along the trigeminal nerve to the brain stem. This is the critical area of the brain pathways, where all the key functions converge. What wasn't said, though quite obvious and pointed out by Patrick Stortebecker of Sweden (of whom more in Chapter 12), is that teeth are also supplied by the trigeminal nerve and dental foci could also track into the cranium and attack central brain tissue in this way.

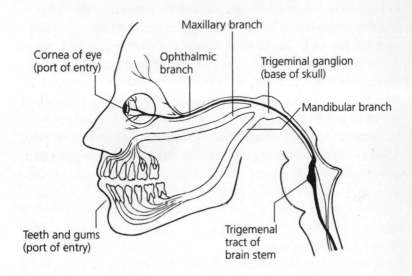

Payling Wright, pathologist at Guy's Hospital in the 1950s, showed the poliomyelitis virus and even inert substances such as ink particles and dyes could travel at a remarkable 2—3 millimetres an hour (5–7 centimetres a day) in this way.[1] Unfortunately, this kind of observation is not given any currency and the vast majority of doctors and medical students do not know of this phenomenon and the appalling health risk it poses.

REMEDY EVALUATION
If the testing system described so far were not enough for a lifetime of work by one man, Voll gave us another gift of technological insight. We call it 'remedy evaluation'. How this came about is ascribed to one of those lucky accidents, a case of the prepared mind being ready at the right place at the right time to be able to benefit from what, to others, would merely be a baffling observation.

Let Voll tell his own story:

> I diagnosed one colleague as having chronic prostatitis and advised him to take a homeopathic preparation called Echinacea 4X. He replied that he had this medication in his office and went to get it. When he returned with the bottle of Echinacea in his hand, I tested the prostate point again and made the discovery that the point reading which was previously up to 90 had decreased to 64, which was an enormous improvement in the prostate value. I had the colleague put the bottle aside and the previous measurement returned. After holding the medication in his hand the measurement value went down to 64 again, and this pattern repeated itself as often as desired.[2]

Voll went on to verify this startling discovery with many other patients and found it to be consistent and very helpful in choosing appropriate treatments.

Thus was remedy evaluation born, though Abrams and Boyd had reported it earlier (Chapter 1) and it was subsequently forgotten.

How It Works

Part of the EAV circuit includes a test plate or a 'honeycomb' – that is, a metal block with slots to take small phials of test substances for comparison. The plate has to be on the passive electrode side of the circuit, so that the remedy 'signal' has passed through the plate and *then* the patient, before being picked up by the probe and completing the loop back to the instrument (See illustration opposite).

If we accept the presence of the Indicator Drop as indicative of a pathological process somewhere along the meridian system, then logically any remedy which removes that drop and restores the reading level will have a beneficial impact. We can put a remedy into the circuit and test the response. If it improves matters somewhat but does not eliminate the adverse read completely, it is open to the practitioner to add other likely therapeutic agents until a satisfactory formula is obtained. Thus we can build a therapeutic regimen with the assurance that it is at least *likely* to work.

Dr Kuo-Gen Chen of the Department of Physics at Soochow University in Taipei has researched medicine testing extensively and explains that 'When a medicine sample is put on the metal plate of the EDS (electro-dermal screening) circuit, the electron waves passing through the plate will be phase modulated. When

Test meter (12 microampere)

Medicine testing honey comb

1" brass bar (hand electrode)

Stylus (pick up elecrode)

these waves later pass through the patient's body, a given signal is transported to the proper organ or tissue by resonant absorption.' In his view, testing is an application of *quantum mechanical quasi phase matching*.[3]

Rapid large-scale testing of remedies can be done by arranging racks of trays containing large numbers of phials. The Dermatron or other sensing device is then connected to each rack in turn; when a rack reads positive, individual trays are tested until the right one is identified; finally each individual phial in this tray can be switched into the circuit until the necessary remedy is located.

In this day and age you would expect computers could help and you would be right. We come to this in Chapter 8.

ALLERGY TESTING

The alert reader will probably quickly deduce the reverse side of this remedy-testing coin: *that it is possible to identify substances which bring about an Indicator Drop where there previously wasn't one and therefore assess them as harmful.* If bringing milk into the picture produces the same Indicator Drop as weedkiller, the therapeutic implications are obvious.

Thus one of the applications of EAV is to look electronically for 'allergies'. After more than two decades of work in the allergy field I can add my own comment here. I have many times observed that patients can become ill without ingesting or breathing their allergens. Sometimes just close proximity to the reagent can do it. In 1987 a young woman from Hong Kong flew over to see me in the UK. Her problem sounded bizarre; but she told it to the right person, because I believed her. Karen Rackham said she felt ill if she was merely in the same room as a cup of tea! It was indeed an allergy and subsequently we were able to help.

Providing the substance comes into the individual's L-Field, it can cause energy disturbance (remember the L-Field extends to infinity but in practice falls away very quickly, according to the inverse square law). Thus there have been many occasions when a highly-sensitive patient has had to be moved to the other side of the test room, away from the racks of testing substances.

I am now convinced that allergy is primarily an information field effect and not a biochemical or humoral one. The neutralizing solutions or vaccines of the Miller method, described in full in my earlier books, are simply another energy medicine dispensation and this explains why putting the neutralizing dose under the person's tongue sometimes works almost instantly. The relief can occur before there is any time for a humoral transfer via the circulatory system. This clinical observation accords very well with the theories of Professor Jacques Benveniste, who holds that all molecules have an electromagnetic information signature which itself can produce the same clinical effect as the molecular substance, even when no chemical is present. He likens it to listening to Pavarotti or Elton John on CD, when the artiste is not actually present.[4]

Naturally, this is highly controversial and regarded as little more than quackery by many doctors. But if one accepts the validity of the Indicator Drop and what it is telling us, this application of electronic allergy testing is at least consistent with the rest of the EAV system.

Is There Any Supportive Proof?

Naturally any scientifically-orientated doctor would want to see some objective proof of what EAV can do. I am pleased therefore on two counts to report two small-scale studies by Julia J. Tsuei and others using EAV to evaluate food allergies and hypertension.

Tsuei received her medical education in China, Taiwan and the US and naturally has a strong affinity for TCM; acupuncture in particular. She has been engaged in several research programmes to further the scientific credibility of acupuncture and Voll's electro-dermal technique.

The food allergy test was simple but sound. Thirty volunteers were used. Allergies identified by the Voll method described above were compared with findings from five other recognized allergy tests: history, skin tests, RAST, IgE levels, and food challenge testing. Voll testing correlated well, particularly with results from challenge tests which, logically at any rate, should tell us the most about food allergy (personally I have strong reservations about the use of food challenge tests as the benchmark in scientific trials).[5]

Tsuei and her team carried out another study on hypertensive patients which is also worth reporting. There were 336 participants, 171 normals and 165 hypertensive individuals. Measurement points were selected based on either TCM or Voll's hypothesized correlations, totalling 56 points tested on each participant.

The 56 points could be divided into seven groups, of which two were measuring cardiovascular energy, three were not, and a further two groups measured both cardio-vascular and non-cardiovascular points. The first group, measuring only cardiovascular energy, correlated extremely well with systolic and diastolic blood pressure, and the other cardio-vascular group also correlated with left-ventricular mass (hypertrophy due to excess blood pressure). Indicator Drops (IDs) on these points gave the most accurate method of identifying the hypertensive patients. But there were also significant relationships between IDs and left-ventricular mass and either systolic or diastolic pressures among three of the five remaining groups.[6]

THE MECHANICS OF EAV

Voll's work was furthered by Professor William A. Tiller of the Department of Material Sciences and Engineering at Stanford University in California. During the 1970s Tiller and other material scientists were investigating the properties of skin to determine the requirements for prosthetic skin, which could be used to treat burns and other skin graft procedures. They studied elasticity, resistance, permeability, chemistry and many other biological properties of skin.

Some researchers, including Tiller, were surprised to find that certain points on the skin had much lower resistance than elsewhere. They knew nothing of Voll's work but soon realized that what they had located were acupuncture points. Tiller studied the dynamics of acupuncture points. The data obtained during these investigations revealed a complex, changing system of information. His model grew to include several electrical properties, such as resistance, conductance and capacitance:

Conductance is the reverse of resistance and measures how well electrons flow.

Capacitance is caused when charge builds up across an electrically resistant barrier; there are several such layers in the skin. All of this means that skin conductivity is far more subtle than just the properties of a wire cable. Many factors play a part, the cells of the different skin layers influencing the diffusion and permeability of electrically-charged ions such as sodium, potassium and chloride ions. Tiller began to refer to acupuncture points as 'windows of information'. According to his model, the health status of the organ in question affects the concentration and diffusion of ions at the points along the meridian, and thus the rate of electron flow, which is what EAV measures.

We need far more studies in this area. Unfortunately, research in the alternative medical field is grossly underfunded. We are lucky, therefore, when an academic institution chances to become interested in this way.

CAUTION

It is very important for the reader or potential patient submitting to EAV to remember one thing, which is that what we are measuring with this system is energetic disturbance. It is *not* equivalent to a blood test or special x-ray, demonstrating gross pathology. We can find the energy signal of cancer of the colon and yet *absolutely nothing can be detectable clinically*. The energetic system is saying that trouble may be coming and be able to characterize what the likely nature of it will be. Obviously there is great preventative potential here. But there are strictly no grounds for disputatious exchanges with conventional doctors or accusations of 'missing' the diagnosis.

This sometimes poses great difficulties for EAV practitioner (many of whom, it must be said, are *not* qualified doctors anyway). A natural desire is present to try to persuade conventional physicians to investigate what has been found energetically and see if there is confirmatory structural or biochemical evidence of disease. But one is inviting ridicule and hostility by revealing one's source of the diagnostic suspicion. Perhaps it is not conceited to hope that the publication of this book will prove helpful when these ticklish situations arise; it could be given to the uninformed physician as a primer.

Casebook: Female, 38 Years

Stan Richardson, a capable if medically-unqualified Voll practitioner in Heckmondwicke, Yorkshire has the following remarkable story to tell:

A woman telephoned one day, asking for help, saying she was sick and frightened she would die. Could Stan help?

When she attended, she looked ghastly and even Stan was concerned. Without allowing her to explain anything, he sat her down and surveyed the initial points. It showed serious drops on the stomach, small intestine and large intestine meridians. Only *then* did he ask her, 'What's been happening?'

She explained that for over three weeks she had been suffering from overwhelming diarrhoea and vomiting. She could keep nothing down. Medicine from the family practitioner was ineffective. She had lost over 3 stone (40 lb) in weight and was frightened but preferred to see an EAV specialist she trusted, rather than attend a hospital.

Stan then resumed and stopped, quite puzzled, when he found a strong resonance that said *rabies* was present in the stressed organs. He didn't tell the patient this but asked the quite reasonable question: 'Have you been abroad lately?' The patient answered that she had just come back from India and been ill ever since she'd arrived home.

'Were you bitten by any animal?' Stan asked; again a very pertinent question. The woman insisted that she had not. Eventually, Stan had to reveal to the patient that the signal from her tissues was rabies. After discussion it emerged that this woman, in her misguided kindness, had been feeding dogs with kitchen scraps at the back door of her hotel in Delhi each night. Clearly what had happened is that she had been licked by a rabid animal and had swallowed the virus from her own fingers, resulting in the appalling intestinal symptoms.

Normally, rabies is spread by a bite which breaks the skin, the virus enters the nerves and travels backwards to the brain, where it is deadly. She had escaped a fatal disease by amazing good luck.

Stan supplied her with a mixture of homeopathic medicines which remedy-testing had said would be beneficial. Her symptoms ceased within 24 hours. By the end of the week she had gained back 10 pounds and eventually made a rapid and full recovery. She had fought, and won, a serious medical battle within her body, using nothing more than quantum energies.

The importance of this illustrative Virtual Medicine story is not merely that it is dramatic and life-saving. It is that *no conventional doctor in his or her right mind would have diagnosed rabies in this situation, or even considered it*. Yet the virtual energy signal showed quite clearly it was present, and with a suitable remedy led the patient back to safety.

Otherwise, she might well have died of severe 'gastro-enteritis', without the hospital doctors ever suspecting what the cause was.

MOTOYAMA AND THE AMI

It would be neglectful to write a chapter describing Voll's work in favourable terms without at least mentioning a similar and contemporaneous development by Tokyo clinical psychologist (also priest, yogi and psychic) Hiroshi Motoyama. His 'Chakra Instrument' has already been discussed on page 40.

Motoyama's AMI system (*Apparatus* for Measuring the Functional Conditions of *Meridians* and their Corresponding *Internal* Organs) is based on the principles of TCM. It was designed to detect organ excess or deficiency by measuring the response to a

3-volt electrical stimulus, sampled at very high frequency. It calculates four different parameters from which the diagnosis is made:

1 autonomic nervous system
2 flow of Ch'i
3 immune system
4 organism's response.

Measurements are taken on the Ting points (end points of meridians) using a double-layer electrode which is totally free of pressure artefacts, unlike Voll's data collection. The clinical information derived is useful, and arguably this system is the most reliable and objective electro-dermal diagnostic test.

Dr Julian Kenyon of the Centre for the Study of Complementary Therapies in Southampton, UK, has carried out a statistical analysis of three machines: the AMI, the segmental electrogram (SEG), from the Vega stable (see Chapter 5) and Kirlian photography. Kenyon dismisses Kirlian photography as worthless, with a co-efficient of variation of over 50 per cent; his own system, the SEG, was 35 per cent and needed to be under 15 per cent ideally. But the AMI returned accuracy at the level of 5–10 per cent (different for each of the above four parameters but all within this excellent range). According to Kenyon, this 'Puts the AMI in a class of its own when compared to other electrodermal diagnostic devices'.[7] What may eventually prove more significant is that the AMI has now been adopted by the Japanese government for official medical screening technology, which is a most satisfactory step forward in Virtual Medicine.

CHAPTER 5

THE VEGATEST

It is said that Reinhold Voll submitted the last few additions to the EAV system a matter of days before his death. Whether this is whimsy or truth, it is clear that he achieved remarkable things despite the blight of a terminal illness. His life work completed, there was little point in going on suffering.

Two subsequent, related developments emerged during the 1970s. Both came into clinical use while Voll was still alive. We shall look at each in some detail in the next two chapters.

The basic problem with Voll's raw method was that it was complex and difficult to organize the data gleaned in a meaningful hierarchical manner. Many points had to be tested and he was gathering *too much* data. It was thus a very laborious and time-consuming procedure which made it exhausting for both the patient and the practitioner.

Starting in the early 1970s Helmut Schimmel hit upon a simple improvement which was to stay with only one testing reference point, usually on the hand for convenience, and introduce diagnostic test ampoules containing low-dose homeopathic extracts of different mammalian organs (usually pig). Applying the same logic to the meaning of an Indicator Drop, if the pathological reading appeared when the liver D4 ampoule was placed in the circuit this would infer problems with the patient's own liver. The test organ ampoule was energetically resonating with the distressed organ tissues within the body. Schimmel called his instrument the Vegetative Test Machine, or Vegatest for short (often just 'Vega').

Again, the core diagnostic indicator is the drop in energy (decrease in measured skin resistance), coupled with a musically falling electronic wail. As with all EAV devices, I find that practitioners tend to test 'by ear', not just by needle deflection. Schimmel named this cadence the *'disorder control'* and it is calibrated at the start of testing by introducing some poison into the 'honeycomb' of the EAV circuit (the test plate – a metal block with slots to take small phials of test substances for comparison – see Figure 7, page 65), such as an ampoule of Paraquat or Lignocaine. It is not easy to master the use of this indicator, but those who can manage it have at their disposal a rapid and approximately accurate means of testing large numbers of organs, pathogens and likely treatments.

PRELIMINARIES

Vega testing is measuring extremely fine energy oscillations, either in the quantum realm or connected with spin phenomena described on page 42, or some unknown mechanism. This makes it highly susceptible to 'noise' and corruption of signals. Proper observance of start-up procedure is therefore important.

The test room must be free from geopathic stress (see page 170). Computers, x-ray machines and other electronic apparatus should be situated well away from the test zone (or at least switched off), making certain there is no interference from equipment in adjacent rooms or even above and below the test room. Electromagnetic fields travel through walls. Even electrical cables give off a substantial magnetic field, and for normal household and commercial voltages the patient must be seated at least 70 cm (2 feet 4 inches) from the nearest power source and at least 1.5 metres (5 feet) from any fluorescent lighting.

It is important that the tester is not personally geopathically stressed, otherwise he or she is likely to 'find' this condition on all patients. In fact if any condition keeps arising in consecutive cases, the first thing the astute BER (bio-energetic resonance) practitioners think of is that they are picking up their own disorder.

The practitioner needs to be in good shape health-wise, and well-rested. Sick patients are often in a predominantly yin phase and tend to drain the practitioner's energies (even lay-people may notice this effect with certain invalids). An exhausted tester cannot get good results. You may notice that the practitioner wears a peculiar magnetic belt. This is said to provide additional protection when testing. Nevertheless, it is unlikely that the practitioner can realistically test for more than a few hours per day without becoming substantially yin and unable to get meaningful results.

CHOOSING THE REFERENCE POINT

Just as in EAV, the Vega specialist tests on an acupuncture point. The tips of the fingers are readily accessible and are chosen by preference: the so-called 'Ting points' just at the corner of the nail bed. The allergy vessel, endocrine or connective tissue meridians are common preferences.

A point has no testing potential unless it can first be made to give off a disorder read, so the practitioner begins by establishing this important pre-requisite. Gentle probing should give a reading around 100 and when a poison is introduced into the metal honeycomb the subsequent reading drops markedly. Ideally, the fall should be 20–30 points on the scale. If this is impossible to obtain, then amplifiers are introduced, in this case ampoules of Epiphysis D30 (30X), until the reading is sufficient to be useful (the homeopathic dilution scale is explained in Chapter 7). The amplifiers are left in the honeycomb throughout the testing session.

Obviously, since the same point is being used over and over, it may well become traumatized and cease to give off any further disorder control. This is especially liable with a beginner using nervous, heavy-handed pressure. Another point has to be selected, but it must be checked for a disorder read before proceeding.

STRESSING THE BODY

It may seem surprising at first, but the body often needs stressing lightly in order to unmask energy disorders. The body's own bioenergetic compensatory mechanisms can be remarkably good at covering up a problem (a reason why normal medical diagnostic skills may be needed as well as an interest in these new methods).

Under normal circumstances the body will always endeavour to obtain a homeostatic balance of the energy flow within the body and the surrounding field. Sometimes only when an additional burden is imposed on the body do masked disturbances become noticeable. Ideally, we would like to choose a mild stressor that produces no harm and is soon re-balanced after testing.

In practice the best approach has been found to be a small electrical shock applied to Lymph 1 and Allergy 1 (points suggested by Voll). A piezo-electric device called a PM 2000 is generally used, which administers a mild charge of 4,000 volts per millisecond. It sounds scary but the current is mild and the patient rarely feels anything at all. Alternatively, the Vega machine also has a 13 Hz provocation output which can by used. This is a stressor frequency (low beta).

The body is thus required to make a compensatory response, which will divert the masking energies and expose real pathological readings which could otherwise be missed.

FINDING THE STRESSED ORGANS

As quickly as possible the Vega tester wants to get to grips with the most stressed organs. This is where the key pathology lies and where the therapeutic response is going to be maximum. This is done by testing a series of organ ampoules, usually at the D4 (4X) potency.

Testing can be speeded up by testing brackets or racks of test ampoules simultaneously. A bar connected by a wire to the honeycomb and laid across several ampoules at once gives a result which is referenced to all those ampoules. If a read appears, then one of the ampoules is active. This can be located by examining them one by one. If the whole bracket is negative, then all of them can be set aside and time has been saved.

The knowledgeable Vega tester will learn to relate what shows up to the patient's clinical condition. It is of course possible that he or she is unaware of any relevant subjective symptoms. Let me once again repeat that the search is for an energetically disturbed organ, which will not necessarily be 'diseased' by the criteria of Western laboratory medicine. We correct the disturbance, Nature does the rest. Only if the energy is left untreated may pathology ensue.

FILTERS

The range and sophistication of the Vega machine is greatly extended by the use of what Schimmel called 'filters', that is, extra ampoules of test reagents introduced into the circuit which modify the response. Reagents have been chosen empirically, and supposedly give further information about organ status and the disease process. For example, here is a list of filters and what they tell us about a disturbed organ:

Zincum met D400	Severe organ stress
Zincum met D200	Most stressed organ
Zincum met D60	Critical organ stress
PhosphorousD32	Most damaged organ
Ars. Alba D60	This is the origin of the patient's complaint

I have already introduced the concept of a focus in the previous chapter. Filtering with the homeopathic remedy Thuja D30 will show a focus is present, and this can be related to the relevant organ. Causticum D60 shows a focus with a disturbance field. There is actually a certain logic to these potencies; thus Causticum D400 (more potent) shows a *dominant* focus with a disturbance field. Generally, the higher the potency that reacts, the more severe the disease.

If the clinical condition is caused by or associated with psychological disorder, a number of emotional filters can clarify matters further. Thalamus D4 will show a neurological disturbance based on autonomic dysfunction. Epiphysis D4 tells us that psychogenic stress is present. Mandragora radice D30 shows exogenous depression, and at the D60 potency tells us it is endogenous in nature. Hypothalamus D800 shows psychosomatic illness; Epiphysis D400 shows hypersensitivity.

Geopathic stress has become a matter of keen interest among alternative practitioners. Chapter 10 investigates aspects of this issue is detail. Meanwhile, the Vega system claims to have filters which can tell us more about a patient's problem:

Geopathic Stress Filters

Silica D60	Geopathic stress present
Iron filings	Geomagnetic stress
Quartz sand	Curry grid
Cuprum met. D800	Double grid stress
Phosphorous D60	Electromagnetic field stress
Agate	Yin stress (discharging field)
Calc. carb. D1	Yang stress (charging field)
Radium bromide D1000	Ionizing radiation exposure
Silica D2000	Frequency stress

Other filters can tell us if the patient is yin- or yang-dominant (linseed oil and sugar water, respectively), mercury toxic (Merc sol. 30), vitamin-deficient (Manganum D200), enzyme-deficient (Zincum met. D200) or hormone-deficient (Molybdenum met. D200).

I have some problem with the nature and efficacy of these 'filters'. They were largely developed by Schimmel and seem very subjective, as well as empirical. However, I do accept that the Staufen pharmacy, which prepares the ampoules, manufactures strictly ethical products, using dilutions of real-time substances to create the filters.

Something is going on, that is clear; I know a case where Radium bromide D1000 read on a woman patient – it emerged her husband worked in the Sellafield Nuclear Power Station. The tester knew nothing of this at the time. Did she carry minute traces of radioactive material? If not, what strange quantum ripple or 'etheric' message was picked up by the woman from her spouse and carried to the practitioner's clinic?

I find these matters fascinating and filled with the richness and luxurious mystery of Nature, rather than an affront to my scientific training. I just think it is high time that proper evaluation studies were carried out and we got past the 'empirical' stage which has now dragged on until one could call it entrenched opinion.

The Vega machine manufacturers are fond of attacking other people's technology. It is time they applied the rules to themselves. What little material is published is mainly in German and this does not advance the international stature of this potentially enlightening test system.

STRESS INDEX

A novel and useful concept, introduced by Dr Erwin Schramm with his Neo Bio-Electronic Test, is that of 'biological age'. It was taken up by Schimmel and also appears in a number of subsequent devices (see page 190). This has nothing to do with calendar age (years) of the test patient but with the vitality and resistance of his or her tissues. The higher the biological age, the more prone the body is to decay and malignant processes. A more descriptive term might be 'stress index'.

Schimmel used potentized embryonic mesenchyme tissue as the reference test agent and gave a range arbitrarily calibrated from 1 to 21. A filter of Cuprum met. D400 is put into the honeycomb. Apart from amplifiers this is the only ampoule used, and it will set the 'disorder control' (see page 74). One by one, starting with 21 and working down, the Mesenchyme ampoules are put in to test; if the Vega reading reverts to 100 (the reference point or pre-requisite of Vega testing, indicating no disorder) this is positive.

Usually testing shows a high age (representing the pathology), a mid-range value (representing the body's present resistance capability) and a low value which is felt to be the 'optimum' biological age for that person.

Reference ranges are shown here:

1–6   These represent the range of normal cellular respiration and do not normally need treatment.

7–10   Indicate pre-clinical phases or functional disturbance with clinically manifest changes.

11–13 Usually clinically recognizable disease.

14–15 The beginning of chronic degenerative changes. Pre-malignant.

16–17 Possible micro-malignancies may be present.

18–21 Possible macro-malignancies which need to be tracked down.

Readings above 10 are usually a sign of clinically manifest disease.

The idea with therapy is to help the patient get down to his or her 'optimum biological age' value. But those who teach the Vega method explain that it is unwise to try to come down to the optimum age too quickly, otherwise unmanageable homeostatic stresses, which decrease the body's ability to recover rather than enhance it, may appear. Gradual improvement may take several sessions and a number of different remedies to drive out the disease signal and attain a suitable biological age.

REMEDY FILTERS

The Vega system obviously includes the capability of remedy testing, along the same lines as Voll's method. Possible remedies will give harmonious balanced readings; unsuitable remedies will create or increase the disorder control.

In fact we can be more refined in this. A number of filters introduced into the honeycomb *prior* to remedy testing will increase the success rate markedly. Thus, for example, filtering with the ampoule Ferrum metallicum D800 will eject remedies which are not going to be *tolerated* by the patient; Ferrum metallicum D26 shows it will be *effective*; and Manganum metallicum D26 shows it will be *compatible* with other remedies selected.

Homeopathic remedies, as you will read in Chapter 7, can sometimes have strong effects on the patient, even when ultimately beneficial. It is important to avoid causing too much unnecessary disturbance, since this rarely assists the true course of healing. This triple bracket of remedy filters is helpful in getting the balance just right.

ORGAN THERAPIES

Voll and Schimmel have given us the concept of 'the most stressed organ' and this has naturally led to new therapeutic regimes. Why treat a pain in the foot if the precipitating cause lies in the liver or adrenals? Obviously, medication to enhance organ function is the logical path. Unfortunately, there is the stigma of patent medicines attached to such an approach (I still remember my mother's 'Little Liver Pills'). The fact is that centuries of herbal lore and specialist healing knowledge go into these compound formulas, which is more than can be said for most of the allopathic medicine range, where treatments come and go like fashions as they are found to be too toxic and then swept under the carpet. The truth remains that there are considerable degrees of lowered function before gross pathology finally appears. It is right to give the body support at *this* stage, not when pathology has finally engulfed the organ. This is so elementary, one wonders why the medical profession has such a struggle with the simple logic involved. Conventional tests for liver function require alterations in blood status or actual anatomical structure before a diagnosis of disease can be made. Yet these changes represent the final *failure* of the body to compensate. Long before that stage, Nature is working hard to keep everything going as it should, a nip here, a tuck there and a little bit of patch and mend. This is hardly optimal, and yet doctors will so often pronounce 'Your blood work is normal, *therefore there is nothing wrong*', when manifestly there *is* a problem and the patient feels unwell. It can be a question of degree.

Here is where energy medicine triumphs because it measures the electrical status of the organ and monitors its function as a whole. One might think of an 'organ gestalt' (whole composite). Subtle changes in this complete electrical field can reflect the fact the several different functions aren't working exactly as they should, while yet there is nothing majorly wrong.

Organ support could include a vitamin and mineral panel, such as my adrenal stress formula, digestive enzyme aids (to boost pancreatic insufficiency) or a liver nutrition formula. This can be combined with physical measures such as a coffee enema to stimulate the liver (common procedure with cancer cases), or colon cleanse where parasites and other bowel toxins are suspected.

SIMPLE LIVER CLEANSE
If you are not getting any results on therapy after three weeks; if you had an initial good result but have started feeling unwell again; or if you have had many years of toxic build-up (drugs, alcohol, tobacco, etc.), you may benefit from a detox programme and a simple liver cleanse.

If you have started a detox programme, this may release further toxins from the fatty and connective tissue where they have been lurking. Sometimes body metabolism can't cope properly at these times and you may go into an overload crisis. Typical signs would include:

- feeling heavily hung-over in the morning, even when you've not been drinking
- slow getting started in the morning
- feeling unduly tired or drained
- having a very low tolerance of alcohol.

There is no need to attempt the extremely heroic 'liver flushes' sometimes in vogue in the alternative field. You may release showers of gallstone gravel but the procedure is potentially dangerous and rather misguided. It overlooks the key principle, that a little push in the right direction will stimulate Nature far more effectively than a shunt with a juggernaut. Instead try this simple formula for 10 days (you can then repeat it a few days each month):

Recipe
- 6 tablespoons of lemon juice
- 3 tablespoons of virgin olive oil (cold pressed)
- 1 small garlic clove, crushed
- Pinch of grated ginger
- Pinch of cayenne pepper

Whisk in a blender and drink immediately. Do not eat for at least 1 hour afterwards.

The acid test, of course, is treating the energetically ailing organ and being able to observe the resultant recovery in health. Whereas no method of testing and treatment is foolproof, the Vegatest approach gives successes often enough to be considered a very valuable attack on the disease process.

PHENOLIC TESTING

A special and very useful application of the Vegatest is that of phenolic testing. I have written about this in my previous book *The Complete Guide to Food Allergy and Environmental Illness*.

In 1979 Dr Robert Gardiner, Professor of Animal Science at Brigham Young University, Utah, began to speculate that his own allergies might be caused by a sensitivity to certain aromatic phenol-based compounds that are found naturally in plant foods and pollens. He acquired some of the pure compounds, made serial dilutions and began to experiment by taking sub-lingual (under the tongue) doses and noting the results.

Sure enough, he found that some phenolic substances reproduced his main symptoms. Not only that, but neutralizing these reactions with subsequent low-dose antidotes of the Miller-method type effectively solved his allergy problems. He was able to eat most foods without reactions. He experienced a major improvement in health.

In other words, allergy to coffee might really be an allergy to chlorogenic acid which is found in the coffee bean. Injecting the chemical produces the same allergic wheal and flare response as the food itself would. There are many such compounds in food. Milk contains 13, tomato has 14, soya 9. A little expertise in these phenol families leads to new allergy diagnostic skills. For example, someone reacting to beef, milk, banana, yeast, potato and tomato might actually be allergic to nicotinic acid. The table below gives a number of common foods and their phenolic content.

PHENOLIC COMPOUNDS IN SOME COMMON FOODS

Compound	Found in
Apiol	almonds, beef, carrot, celery, cheese, milk, oranges, peas, rice, soya beans
Capsaicin	milk, onion, potato, tomato
Cinnamic acid	apple, banana, beet sugar, celery, cheese, grapes, lettuce, milk, onion, oranges, peas, tomato
Coumarin	apple, banana, beef, cane sugar, carrot, celery, cheese, chicken, egg, lamb, lettuce, oranges, peas, potato, rice, soya beans, tomato, wheat, yeast
Eugenol	almonds, beef, carrot, celery, cheese, milk, oranges, peas, soya beans, tomato
Gallic acid	almonds, apple, beet sugar, cabbage, cane sugar, carrot, celery, cheese, egg, grapes, lettuce, milk, onion, oranges, peas, potato, tomato, wheat
Malvin	apple, cabbage, carrot, celery, chicken, egg, grapes, lamb, lettuce, milk, onion, soya beans, tomato
Menadione	apple, celery, egg, grapes, lettuce, onion, peas
Nicotine	beef, milk, potato, tomato, yeast
Phenyl isothiocyanate	beef, cabbage, chicken, egg, lamb, milk, onion, peas, soya beans, tomato
Phlorizin or phloridzin	apple, beef, beet sugar, cheese, egg, grapes, lamb, lettuce, milk, orange, soya bean, yeast
Piperine	beef, beet sugar, cheese, chicken, grapes, lamb, milk, onion, peas, potato, soya beans, tomato, yeast

Piperonal	almond, beef, beet sugar, cabbage, lamb, lettuce, milk, tomato, yeast
Rutin (quercitin)	apple, beef, beet sugar, cane sugar, carrot, celery, cheese, chicken, egg, grapes, lamb, lettuce, milk, orange, pea, potato, rice, soya beans, tomato, wheat, yeast
Vanillylamine	almonds, apple, beef, cheese, grapes, lamb, lettuce, milk, onion, orange, potato, soya beans, tomato, yeast

The story was taken up by Dr Abram Ber, who began testing patients for sensitivity of this type with a Dermatron. He was able to claim success with a wide diversity of complaints, particularly in infants and children, getting excellent results with autism, dyslexia, insomnia, enuresis, respiratory allergies, abdominal pains and asthma. In adults, remissions were achieved with many chronic problems such as migraine, fatigue, depression, asthma, arthritis, colitis, hypertension, menstrual problems, skin diseases, chronic constipation and cardiac arrhythmias.

People struggling against their allergies suddenly found a whole new dimension of management for their condition. This can rightly be ascribed as a major benefit of the Vegatest system, or any EAV derivative. Intradermal testing of these compounds would be slow, painful and time-consuming. The Vegatest is quicker, non-invasive and far cheaper to administer than hours of intradermal tests, though as someone who has done both I believe it is not as accurate and is subject to the cautions discussed in the following section on objectivity ('Considerations', below).

Some phenolic compounds have been found to correlate well with certain diseases. Cinnamic acid (in fruits, cheese and nuts) is a major cause of skin irritation in eczema and other dermatological conditions; coumarin (wheat, rice, barley, corn, soya, cheese, beef and eggs) contributes significantly to arthritis; malvin (found in some 35 common foods, including chicken, egg, corn, milk and soya bean) may be associated with autism, dyslexia, learning difficulties, epilepsy and other neurological disorders in children.

There are many other phenol-based compounds which are crucial to our physiology, such as neurotransmitters (serotonin is one), hormones, co-enzymes and pharmacological food ingredients such as caffeine, enzyme inhibitors and anti-nutrients.

The Vegatest is used to establish neutralizing dilutions in just the same manner that any remedy testing is carried out. The ideal antidote would be that which eliminates the disorder read when an allergy filter is in the honeycomb. The patient takes these neutralizing dilutions sub-lingually for a month and then returns for re-testing. The aim is to get down to the first dilution (5X), meaning that the patient has become fairly tolerant of the allergen. He or she can then use a weekly or twice-weekly maintenance dose.

CONSIDERATIONS

The Psychokinetic Effect

Vega testing requires more skill than EAV but both are difficult to perform well. The clumsy Vega probe is certainly part of the problem. I myself learned to use this technique in the 1980s and it would not be right to withhold from the reader that the machine tends to give the practitioner what he or she expects. In other words, I liken it to 'electronic dowsing'. Those who watched Schimmel himself at work observed that he often varied his probe pressure and seemed to know what he was going to 'discover' before he found it.

This raises the question that the disorder control (or indeed Voll's Indicator Drop for that matter) are no more than subconscious muscle responses to a preconceived mental intuition. In a world of supposed objective science, this standard of testing may seem a little strange; it may not sit comfortably for some. Therefore it is vital to make clear to the reader that any such 'objectivity' is a myth. No scientific study has ever been devised which eliminates the element of operator intrusion. This is one of the main things that quantum physics has taught us.

Dutch worker Van Wijk investigated this further in 1989.[1] He carried out studies on EAV performance. Voll's method of point testing was addressed in great detail and it was found that a pressure of 125 grammes was optimum. At this level the variability of resistance was less than 5 per cent. The average recovery rate of refractory skin tissue at this optimum pressure was 10 seconds. Van Wijk really showed that changes in conductivity are pressure-sensitive and independent of electrical current which, on the face of it, undermines Voll's work.

However, in 1992 Van Wijk showed that trained practitioners could identify an 'active' ampoule among 19 blanks over 90 per cent of the time (1:20 probability).[2] This is a far higher rate than chance and considerably better than conventional medicine recovery rates. The inference, therefore, is that skilled EAV practitioners will benefit their patients most of the time. But it may be no more than a subtle form of muscle testing (kinesiology).

In fairness, leading Vegatest practitioner Dr Julian Kenyon acknowledges the inevitable inclusion of the psychokinetic effect and defends it heavily. As he says, 'It is important to recognize the part played by the practitioner in bio-energetic regulatory techniques such as the Vegatest method. This does not detract from their validity but merely means that the Vegatest and similar methods are looked at for what they are, no more and no less. They are however easier to carry out than using a totally psychic effect such as in dowsing because an objective subtle electrical change is taking place.'[3]

The Human Detector

My own view is that the human organism is capable of operating as a sensitive quantum bio-magnetic detector and that the results are at least in a degree objective. In other words the tests can be blind and the operator will sense something; that 'something' will lead to a subconscious alteration in probe pressure. I judge this valid scientifically. However, a great deal more investigative work needs to be done, otherwise all this is food for the critics. It does not serve the cause of advancement to duck the awkward issues. Instead we need to address them conscientiously and vigorously.

The necessary mind—brain link probably comes within known physics laws which at present remain hidden from view simply because of current practical limitations and gaps in our theoretical understanding (as was the case for so many centuries regarding the body's energy fields). All we can say with our present state of knowledge is that a thought potential somehow excites an electromagnetic response which can then act at a distance.

We have already seen that the human energy field can damage or disrupt computers, watches and other sensitive electronic equipment. I wrote about this in *The Allergy Handbook* and suggested that allergy sufferers seemed to have far more powerful electromagnetic 'auras' than most people. As a spectacular demonstration of this human energy charge, an experiment was conducted at the Menninger Foundation.[4] Exceptional subjects were suspended in front of a large wired copper wall and were shown to give off very substantial electromagnetic fields. These fields were easily capable of disrupting micro-electronics and therefore capable of attracting reads on an EAV instrument.

A cadre of scientists have taken the view that if quantum theory is the best explanation of reality we have at present, then it should take account of mind and consciousness and the part these play in phenomena. Professor D. F. Lawden at Aston University, Birmingham, England, is among those who think that systems which are dependent on the observer state, that is which include consciousness in the nature of the construct, are especially worthy of study.

Several of the Virtual Medicine diagnostic and therapeutic techniques I have detailed in this book are just such examples of psycho-physical states displaying quantum characteristics. Lawden has gone so far as to draw up modifications of the basic equations of quantum mechanics, to allow for possible disturbing psychic effects being introduced by the participants.[5] This has also helped to clarify what constraints to 'reality' there may be, when recognizing there is no absolute or autonomous state. In this, Lawden likens quantum science to the philosophy of Irish bishop George Berkeley (1685–1753), one of the so-called British Empiricists. Berkeley's basic premise was that all matter and material form has no meaning whatever outside the mind. It might be there, but how could we ever contact it without a mind being involved in doing so?

To accept Lawden's argument is effectively to turn scientific thinking on its head. His revision would put ideas and sensations as the primary events, and matter (particles, energy) as secondary participants; this is exactly where our Eastern forebears left our cosmos 4,000 years ago. We have gone through the convolutions of supposedly superior scientific method, right up to the minute and beyond, only to end up where intuitive gifts and metaphysical *knowing* took us a long time ago!

Casebook: Male, 40 Years

Finally, in case this review of objectivity should have suggested that the Vega test or any EAV is of doubtful worth, let me cite a case from the files of world-class EAV specialist Anthony Scott-Morley of Poole in Dorset.

The patient had complained of persistent discomfort in the region of the liver. Routine laboratory examinations by the family doctor had revealed no abnormality. Orthodox treatment including anxiolytic drugs had, not surprisingly, failed. The private opinion of the referring doctor was that the patient was neurotic and would benefit from psychotherapy.

Vega testing showed a stressed liver which was balanced by the ampoule *aflatoxin*. Aflatoxin is a highly toxic fungus commonly growing on mouldy nuts, especially peanuts. Scott-Morley asked the patient if peanuts had any significance for him. The patient expressed great surprise and started to cry.

It emerged that he had been employed as a truck driver and had some months earlier transported a truckload of peanuts to England. On arrival at Customs the consignment had been condemned as mouldy and unfit for human consumption. Yet the driver had, not unnaturally, consumed many handfuls on his journey across Europe.

Treatment using the Aflaxotin nosode resulted in prompt and permanent relief of all symptoms. Conventional medicine could not have mad this diagnosis.

CHAPTER 6

BIORESONANCE THERAPY

We have considered so far how the patient's energy field is paramount, and how disturbances in that field may give rise to disease. A novel idea which evolved in the 1970s, piggy-backing new technological possibilities, was to use modifications of the patient's *own* energy emissions as a means of eliminating disharmony and morbidity. If we can somehow use electronic machines to strengthen the healthy energies and at the same time eliminate the unhealthy ones, whole new therapeutic possibilities open up. This was the line taken by Dr Franz Morell and led along a parallel development sequence to the Vegatest.

The term 'bioresonance therapy' (BRT) has come to mean therapy with the patient's own oscillations. This differs somewhat from the EAV approach on two main counts: first, that one need not identify the cause of pathological oscillations, and second that the counter-agent or means of eliminating the wrong energies need not be some exterior agent, such as a medicine, but can be accomplished by means of modulating or cancelling the unwanted signal, while at the same time strengthening the 'good' energies. We could introduce the term *electronic homeopathy* for this class of healing.

ELECTROMAGNETIC SIGNALS

Pathological electromagnetic oscillations are active alongside normal oscillations in the body of every patient. Indeed, even healthy individuals certainly have some element of such disharmony but, as Lakhovsky suggested, if the energies of the normal cells are stronger than the pathological energies, then health can be maintained (page 21). On the other hand, if Lakhovsky's 'war of energies' goes ill for the tissues and cells, the resulting disturbance of the dynamic equilibrium will lead to disease, even cancer and death. The important point is that the electromagnetic signals from a diseased patient contain all the information needed for therapy, if only we could successfully decode it.

Morell's idea was that we do not necessarily need to decode it, if only we can identify which signals are the problem. Ideally there would be some kind of filtering process to divert the pathological energies, which could then be altered and used to modulate the disease process. The problem is to know which are the bad energies, among the huge volume of information traffic and 'noise' going on round a living organism such as a human body. Fortunately, harmonious energies do tend to be similar from person to person. These are the dynamic energies. Any impinging signal which is fixed is very likely to be non-biological in nature; in other words, harmful.

THE MORA MACHINE

Morell went to work, with his son-in-law Erich Rasche, and together they developed a device now known as the MORA machine (MO from Morell and RA from Rasche). Rasche, an electronics engineer, reports that it was some time during 1976 that Morell handed him over 500 small metal washers. These were colour-coded and, according to Morell, had the 'information signal' imprinted in them of homeopathic potencies. The idea was to use these for remedy testing, along the lines of EAV. Plexiglas sheets holding 100 washers each were made; 10 such sheets would store 1,000 remedy tests.

In fact, nothing directly came of this idea and it was not until the advent of computer technology a decade later that this dream of storing a large number of 'information signals' came to fruition.[1]

However, this got the two men started on research and development, together with bio-physicist Ludger Mersmann, and what they came up with in 1977 was a machine which certainly changed the face of future medicine. We are still only two decades into its development, and so it has far from fulfilled its potential yet. But, scientifically speaking, the principle is simple and sound; technologically it is straightforward; and therapeutically it has proved its usefulness time and time again. As the energy medicine paradigm advances, the MORA machine will grow in stature. Already there are a number of copycat and derivative devices, including the BICOM, which is discussed later.

What the MORA machine basically does is enhance harmonious oscillations to help the tissues overthrow the noxious process, and inverts pathological signals, which effectively cancels them out.

A little more physics is needed here. A wave form has peaks and troughs, as the signal 'oscillates' or varies in intensity. To invert a signal means to put peaks where there were troughs, and vice versa; this effectively results in zero energy, since one cancels out the other (see illustration below). It is very simple to arrange this electronic process. In fact Rasche also arranged that all signals could be passed through to the patient, unaltered; the harmonious signals could be amplified (but would not, logically, be inverted), or the harmonious energy, combined with inverted pathological energy, could both be amplified if necessary.

The input signals from the patient are picked up directly from electrodes held in the hand, or from foot-plates. These are delivered to the machine and modified in various ways. The resulting output or therapeutic signals can be 'played back' through the same electrodes, or via a probe. As in 'Basic Therapy' described below, the input signal may even be taken from a little of the patient's body fluid, such as saliva or blood.

In addition to the electronic apparatus necessary to make these arrangements, the MORA machine is also fitted with an EAV device, since practitioners of BRT are almost invariably involved with EAV, so close are the two disciplines.

However it should be pointed out that the MORA machine probably has more in common with Abrams' Oscilloclast and Boyd's Emanometer than with EAV.[2] Other possibilities offered by this family of machines include the use of low light frequencies, filtered and modulated, which are then played back electronically through skin electrodes, or the use of direct light enhancement (compare this with the machine described in Chapter 9).

A USEFUL EXPERIMENT

Experiments on animals can be revealing. One uses animals not only because doing so throws up fewer moral implications, but also because in doing so one can exclude likely psychological factors.

In a 1985 study using Syrian hamsters, benefits from bioresonance were clearly seen which could have no placebo basis. One group of hamsters was treated with bioresonance, while the controls were left untreated. All other factors, such as food, heat and lighting were kept constant. Various parameters were studied, including red cell count, a differential leukocyte count (thus giving lymphocyte totals), weight and quantitative food hoarding.

The treated group became more lively, their defence and flight reactions were faster and their coats were smoother than those of the controls. Food hoarding, a species sign of health, was considerably higher in the treated group than in the controls.

Among the haematological parameters tested which were significant, the treated group showed a marked rise in lymphocytes, which is equivalent to an increase in immune function and longevity.[3] The protocol, though simple, was impeccable and the results convincing.

Veterinary bioresonance has since become a reality. Animals are said to be particularly rewarding and responsive subjects. It is just as effective with very large animals, as with smaller species. The only difficult group are the very hairy patients!

BASIC THERAPY

The methodology of BRT is relatively simple. Before starting with a therapeutic regimen using a device such as the MORA machine, it is customary to carry out a pre-treatment or so-called 'Basic Therapy'. This means to enhance harmonious energies and invert pathological ones, so strengthening the patient's resources. This can be very important with chronically sick and weakened patients, who want to be in good shape to receive the main therapeutic energies without being knocked over by them!

The patient provides a little saliva which is put into the metal beaker on the input side. This beaker is in effect a receiving device, rather like a radio aerial; the signal is led away through a lead, to be amplified and modulated within the apparatus. Other 'input' samples could include skin scrapings, nasal secretions or vaginal and rectal swabs – in fact any bodily tissue or fluid.

Settings on the machine allow simple choices such as amplification, inversion and filtering. For children it may even be desirable to attenuate the signal somewhat. A few minutes of this pre-treatment is all that is required.

VOLL MERIDIANS

The MORA specialist then goes on to test individual meridians, keeping a note of the readings at each Central Measurement

Point (CMP). This is much in line with Voll's method; balance is taken to be anything between 45 and 55. Again, too high is inflammatory and too low means degeneration. Indicator Drops (IDs) are seen, exactly as you would expect.

But here is where bioresonance enters. With bioresonance it is possible to alter the emanations being collected by the probe at each main pathology point (most abnormal reading or biggest ID), using the amplification, inversion and broadcast principle. The modern MORA has various settings which allow the practitioner to focus on different bands or 'windows' of frequencies. He can then take the incoming signal and make three basic changes: amplify it; invert it and amplify it; or filter out the pathological signals. The way this is decided in practice is by playing each modulation in turn and seeing which brings the point back *nearest* to the ideal 50.

A treatment would then consist of playing the therapeutic signal through the patient for several minutes. The body cannot respond well to the intensity of a constant signal; it becomes refractory. Instead the therapeutic message is broken up into parcels. A fixed number of timed units can be spaced out with pauses between. Empirical tests indicate that 3 seconds of signal followed by 1 second of pause is probably optimum. In this way the full treatment energy is received without resistance by the tissues.

Scorch Marks

At the time of writing I do not use a MORA device, but leading British EAV specialist Stan Richardson has remarked to me that after a BRT session it is often possible to see scorched hand prints on the pickup and output electrode bars. This is especially noticeable if the bars are left untouched overnight and allowed to 'develop' photographically. Moreover, the output side has a different pattern to the input side. Stan feels that there may be some kind of coded message here, if only we could decipher it, akin to the Kirlian photograph (page 47).

This also brings to mind Lakhovsky's theories of cellular radiation and the 'spontaneous radiographs' of C Nodon (page 22).

ALLERGIES

One unusual aspect of the MORA machine, not shared by other EAV apparatus, is the ability to modify allergy signals. I have always argued that allergy is basically an information-field signal, rather than a biochemical process, as explained on page 66. Because of this little-known fact (i.e. that allergy is basically an information-field signal) there is the potential to modify the patient's receptivity to the harmful energy of an allergen.

This is also, incidentally, a good demonstration for those who remain sceptical about the whole process now being described. If the patient's allergen is placed in the beaker and the signal therefrom is played back electromagnctically through the output electrodes, the patient may experience symptoms. It is remarkable that the signal for wheat can provoke, say, an attack of wheezing in an asthmatic. If not, turning up the amplitude of the signal is very likely to do so. This verifies the existence of the allergy and proves that it is *not* a biochemical or immune process, whatever conventional medicine says. It allows us to show once and for all that every substance has a unique energetic signal and that this can harmfully interact with our endogenous energies. No chemical or fluid changes position or enters the patient's body, yet symptoms are triggered!

Treatment of allergies may be effectively carried out by inverting the input signal. It is not easy to see the logic of this but it does seem to work; indeed, in my opinion it is one of the best available uses of the MORA family of devices. Perhaps the body is being electromagnetically reprogrammed using the 'anti-allergy' signal, which can then be incorporated into the energetic dynamics. Treatment takes placc wcckly, with gradually increasing numbers of timed units, rather like the old immunological allergy protection known as hypo-sensitization, where the dose increases until the body can learn to tolerate it. From then on it protects the body in much the same way that any antidote would.

As an amusing aside, this process can be carried out on other substances. If cheap rough whisky or wine is placed into the tray, and then signals from it are inverted and played back *into the bottle*, the resulting drink is unquestionably enhanced. This claim never fails to attract laughter and disbelief from audiences; yet even the most incredulous of sceptics is usually impressed by the happy result. Blind tastings show that there is indeed a difference.

MERCURY AMALGAM

So much has been said about mercury toxicity from dental amalgams that it would be superfluous to debate the issue here. More is said about it in Chapter 12, along with other more important and up-to-the-minute theories.

MORA therapy does offer a new approach to this problem. Whereas one should remove fillings and so eliminate the source of contamination, this does not remove established tissue deposits, which are often considerable. One can try to use chelation agents such as DMPS (dimercapto-propane sulphonic acid) and DMSA (dimercaptosuccinic acid), which bind with the mercury and so eliminate it through the kidneys. But even this has potential dangers, since DMPS actually binds with neurological tissue and so cannot eliminate brain deposits. A better plan is to use the MORA playback facility to invert and counter the mercury signal, in much the same way as is done with an allergen. Rasche claims that this actually enhances the excretion of amalgam compounds.

The EAV part of the device can be used to establish exactly what heavy metal burden is present in the patient's body. This can then be used in the input beaker and the signal inverted, amplified and thus neutralized. Generally, Rasche recommends that the heavier the mercury burden, the higher the amplification needed. This seems to be logically sound.

Treatments are carried out twice a week for 3 to 4 weeks. Drinking copious soft water helps the ion elimination process and this is mainly effective at the time of therapy. In Rasche's words 'The excretion process continues until the earth's natural magnetic field realigns the elementary particles of the remaining amalgam.'[4]

OTHER APPLICATIONS

There are clearly very many possible applications for this energetic approach to health. Some which have had particularly gratifying results include infertility, where sperm count and motility have been seen to increase markedly after BRT; extensive burns, where non-invasiveness is a strong point; healing of bones; eye problems; tinnitus and gynaecological problems. Children appreciate this treatment modality, since no pain is felt and their natural apprehensiveness is soon appeased. The child or infant can sit happily on his or her parent's lap while therapy is administered. ECG electrodes (the kind with rubber elastic straps) can be adapted as electrodes for very small babies.

Bioresonance therapy is especially useful in the management of addictions, such as tobacco and drugs. It is very helpful to an individual going through the unpleasant withdrawal phase to have harmful energies filtered out and natural, health-boosting frequencies amplified. Obviously this does not eliminate the need for the patient to make a clear and determined decision to *stop* indulging their addiction. But by forcing the excretion of toxins and balancing yin-yang energies, the misery is much reduced.

Thus, after a general Basic Therapy, the addictive substance is placed in the input beaker and passed to the patient inverted and amplified, exactly as described for allergens and toxins above. It is essential to prescribe a simultaneous forced excretion therapy, including copious amounts of water, teas, enemas and liver cleansing. Vigorous exercise, lymph massage and depuration saunas are also helpful where possible. Homeopathic drainage support and organ stimulants may also be indicated (see Chapter 7).

Finally, an aggressive vitamin and mineral programme is required, to help the body nutritionally overcome the toxins present and to ensure renewed healing and tissue repair. Withdrawal symptoms are very stressful to the organism and adrenal cortical function is often at maximum revs. High doses of vitamin C in the 10–20 grammes range are also useful as a short-term detoxicant.

Even where the regime proves quickly successful, it is recommended that the patient attends regularly for many months, to reinforce the determination to quit.

PAIN

'Pain is the cry of connective tissue caused by blocked energy'; so the saying goes. This maxim of Dr Weichel was often quoted by Voll. It emphasizes that pain is not really a local manifestation, even though the triggers may appear to be. Morell found benefit from treating the ends of those meridians (Ting points) which pass through the pain area, starting with the mirror-image points on the side opposite the painful area.

This can be followed by picking up signals from the pain area and, after inversion, playing these back to the tissues somewhat distal to the disease area. *Increasing the amplitude of the inverted signal effectively pushes it deeper and deeper into the tissues.*

If pain is intensified during the treatment, this may not be a reason to stop the therapy. The practitioner must decide each case individually, but there can be a degree of beneficial intensification before the pain finally eases off. Sometimes physiological changes can be seen in the skin, such as a white patch becoming visible. This area should be made the target of output therapeutic energies. Treatment is continued until the skin resumes normal colouration.

Casebook: Male, 6 Years

This boy developed an astrocytoma, which has a very bleak prognosis. The consultant neurosurgeon had recommended chemotherapy. The parents, who were Buddhists, had rejected the idea and decided their child would die gently and with dignity, if that was to be. They prayed. Even better, they also took him to see a MORA therapist.

By this time the boy was in a desperate state and was so weak and wasted he had to be helped to walk into the clinic. The practitioner took blood and subjected it to the inversion and amplification process described; just a few minutes for the first visit. The child was sent home with homeopathic support therapy along the lines described for mesenchyme therapy in Chapter 7. Then, by gradually building up the timed units of treatment, once a week and then, eventually, once a fortnight, the lad was soon feeling well. A few months later he was able to resume athletics and playing rugby football.

The practitioner, who could also use a Vega machine, tested and found no remaining tumour signal, but there was a focus which was cystic. At about this time, the parents (without telling the MORA practitioner) took their son back to the original consultant. He was surprised to even see the boy alive. As is often the attitude, he was dismissive and said 'We must have been mistaken in our diagnosis.' This angered the parents, who were naturally incensed at the idea of their son being subject to chemotherapy based on a shaky diagnosis. But the old scans were brought out and re-examined: there could be no doubt. It was a tumour all right. With persuasion, the parents allowed a re-scan which showed that only a cyst now remained where once the tumour had been. The MORA practitioner has a copy of the letter from the hospital confirming this in his files.

This was a very satisfactory result for Virtual Medicine. Incidentally, the specialist never asked what the miraculous treatment was or showed the slightest interest in learning about it. He goes on giving chemotherapy to his patients.

BAND PASS DEVICES

Certain improvements in the basic MORA procedure suggest themselves. A competitive device, developed by former US MORA representative Hans Brügemann, addresses some of the issues. It has taken advantage of available computer technology and is accordingly dubbed the BICOM (BI-ological COM-puter).

It has around a thousand pre-programmed case handlings, with pre-set frequencies and timed units based on the pooled knowledge of many practitioners of the MORA school. Among the problems which can be dealt with in this easy way are:

Problem	Pre-set Programme
eye inflammation	(520)
bladder irritation	(490)
diabetes	(45)
muscular pain	(630)
hacking cough	(540)
wound healing, stimulating	(931)
selenium metabolism, stimulating	(804)
and so on...	

101 is the so-called 'basic programme'. A BICOM practitioner is also offered the possibility of entering and storing their own favourite programmes. This is certainly an advance over the 'manual programming' of the MORA machine and an obvious benefit of computer technology that lends itself to the situation.

But the chief technological advance the BICOM boasts is the use of a *band pass*, a cyclical passage of a narrow 'information window' up and down the scale from 10 Hz to 150,000 Hz. This innovation is based on the observation over many years that therapy works best if oscillations are returned in a relatively narrow range. Otherwise the cellular dynamics may be given too much to deal with.

Couple this with the discovery by Cyril Smith at Salford University, England, that effective bioresonance therapy results in an immediate response, whereas less appropriate or detrimental energies take some time to develop the adverse effect. It makes sense to move rapidly over the ground and give short bursts of therapeutic signals, rather than linger as with the older method.

Thus we have a number of new options in the BICOM, over and above returning all frequencies simultaneously:

1 Only a small part of the frequency is returned, in a selected range, usually chosen by the operator.
2 A range of frequencies is swept just either side of a central set figure. Technically this is known as 'wobble'. The amount of wobble can be varied but still operates within a relatively narrow range.

3 The whole end-to-end range is swept automatically, concentrating on one part at a time, but covering every possible allowed frequency.

It will be seen that only option 3 actually covers all possible frequencies, though not all at once. It may be important to operate over the whole range; since no frequency is transmitted for long the chance of developing adverse effects is almost zero, whereas the benefits, as Smith showed, happen almost instantly. Furthermore, the patient may respond favourably to several different frequencies; in fact commonly does. This ensures these secondary beneficial zones will be visited too; and yet overall it saves the operator time.

A Brief Critique

Much controversy has surrounded the BICOM, some of which, if valid, should rightly be aimed at the MORA machine too. Part of the attack on the BICOM's performance has come from rival manufacturers, such as Vega. The latter claim to have special electronic sensing equipment which has examined the output from the BICOM and shown it to be worthless and not what is claimed. Perhaps this should be seen mainly in terms of a marketing offensive, rather than the purest of scientific motives.

One thing is certainly true: BICOM comes under the anti-radionics legislation in the US and cannot legally be sold there. The American public, it seems, needs protecting from funny waves, even though the US Food and Drug Administration claims these waves are not there!

The EAV device incorporated in the BICOM is perfectly straightforward and cannot be challenged legitimately by Vega. Also the inversion and amplification channels are simple and unarguable electronics manipulations.

The logic and empirical science behind the band pass is perfectly cogent to me. It is notable in this respect that the MORA people have responded by introducing the band-pass facility into their own latest machine.

It is only the pre-programme facility of the BICOM that can be separated from the other aspects and targeted for special criticism. I doubt it is so important, since most BRT practitioners have their own views on suitable treatment programmes.

My own unease comes from the performance of the filter or separator, which is absolutely critical to BRT. If your filter lets through the harmful oscillations, the theory is lost. We have no standard against which to judge what is a pathological signal. I indicated above that any fixed vibration is unlikely to be physiological in nature, but other than that it is little more than speculation what a disease oscillation behaves like. Brügemann defends his separator vociferously by pointing to an experiment which showed that temperature drop in healthy patients, caused by subjecting them to the information signal of mercury in the input beaker, was effectively blocked by it. Without the protection of first passing the signal through the separator, subjects experienced an alarming fall in temperature of almost 2 degrees Centigrade within 30 seconds; the experiment had to be discontinued because of heart fibrillations.[5]

My own view is that such an experiment is grossly unethical if you believe your own story about negative oscillations. But it also seems to me that Brügemann fails to make his scientific point, since this only shows that the machine can single out mercury signals. It does *not* show it is capable of discerning all good from bad among the huge totality of ultrafine oscillations of the body, as is claimed. *What it does show, which is helpful for my text, is that energy signature oscillations of toxic substances have great impact on biological systems*, exactly as Jacques Benveniste believes (see page 112).

Until the manufacturers stop hiding behind proprietary secrets and tell us what they are using in the separator, we cannot properly evaluate their ideas. Perhaps time and further research will clarify matters for us all.

RESISTANCE TO BRT
A number of factors are recognized to impair or block the benefits of BRT. These have been observed empirically over the years and form a basic list of resistance factors to any kind of therapy.

1 The place of therapy is geopathically stressed.
2 The patient's home or workplace is geopathically stressed.
3 There is a tooth focus or strong amalgam stress (see Chapter 12).
4 There are hidden psychological factors preventing success, which would include the practitioner's own doubts or scepticism.
5 There is a nutritional deficiency (*no* therapy works well in the present of nutrient deficiency).
6 There are hidden toxins, parasites or allergies present.
7 Allopathic drugs have a blocking effect. Even alternative therapies can sometimes interfere with each other.
8 The cables are damaged or the electrodes are not cleaned properly (energy disturbance can be carried over from the previous patient).
9 There is interfering scar tissue.
10 The therapist is insufficiently skilled or knowledgeable at what he or she is attempting.

SUMMARY OF BIORESONANCE THERAPY

Hans Brügemann of the Brügemann Institute, which manufactures the BICOM machine, has nicely summarized the chief precepts for understanding bioresonance therapy. In conclusion I give here a modified description of these:

1 In and around the human body there are electromagnetic oscillations. These oscillations are superordinate to the biochemical processes going on in the tissues and are the real control mechanism of tissue function.
2 As well as physiological oscillations there are also pathological interfering oscillations in every person, caused by toxin overload, injury, infection, unresolved disease processes and psychologically negative states (so-called emotional toxins).
3 Both natural and pathological oscillations can be picked up from the skin surface (antenna effect) and led to a suitably tuned therapeutic device.

4 The mixed oscillations from the patient can be modulated in three main ways: (i) healthy signals amplified; (ii) pathological signals inverted (and thus cancelled out); and (iii) filtered, to separate the desirable frequencies from the pathological ones (the latter are, of course, eliminated in this process).

5 No technologically-generated artificial frequencies are needed; only oscillations from the patient which have been modified as given in 4. The basic aim is to strengthen the good oscillations and eliminate the unwanted ones.

6 The body takes its cue from the modulated therapeutic signals and continues to produce enhanced physiological signals and appears to reprogramme itself, so that in future a renewal of the pathological signals is guarded against. Thus the treated harmonious levels of electromagnetic energy go beyond the merely temporary stage of treatment sessions.

7 Beneficial changes in the energy field are followed by a subsequent modification and improvement in biochemical function and physical structure.

8 BRT is successful when the body's own endogenous regulatory forces reassert control and lead to normalization and maintained health.

CHAPTER 7

BASIC TREATMENT MODALITIES

It is time now to consider the medicinal therapy which is integral with EAV and its derivative, computer electro-dermal screening technology (see Chapter 8). In general this type of therapy is based on bio-information and energy; these therapeutic substances could therefore be termed 'Virtual Medicines' in line with our overall theme.

To understand the place of this remarkable form of treatment it is useful to look at a categorization of different forms of therapy:

1 **Invasive Methods**
   Surgery, lasers, moxa therapy
2 **Biochemical Methods**
   a. Inorganic (e.g. minerals)
   b. Organic (e.g. herbs, drugs, vitamins)
3 **Energy Methods**
   Electro-magnetic waves, Reiki, acupuncture,
    bio-magnetism, sound, music, colour therapy, homaccords
4 **Information Methods**
   High-potency homeopathy, Bach flower remedies,
   gem therapy, electrical bioresonance, nosodes and sarcodes.

THE ELEMENTS OF HOMEOPATHY

Almost all practitioners of EAV use what is known as complex homeopathy. To understand its precise advantages it is necessary first to clarify the basic nature of homeopathy. Today it is largely forgotten that this was once a major system of treatment taught in over 25 per cent of US medical schools and that, until the arrival earlier this century of patentable allopathic drugs which could be marketed for huge profits, it enjoyed a sound reputation and was widely practised, both in Europe and the New World.

With the coming of the drug boom, however, there emerged a new supposedly scientific paradigm based on laboratory testing on animals and clinical trials, particularly the double-blind sort. Alternative methods, or more traditional (older) approaches, were re-evaluated as 'not scientific'. Even simple remedies such as good food and rest were more or less rubbished in the stampede for newer and better 'magic bullets'. The attitude which today pervades conventional medicine is that what the treatment of disease needs is something to oppose or crush the unruly process. There is no concept of nurture or helping Nature to perform the cure. Indeed, Nature's generous wisdom is often abused or over-ridden, as in the case of chemotherapy or commando surgery for cancer.

Even less do many modern doctors understand that the disease process is necessary; it is a natural complement to the exigencies of life. Without the fight-back response, or what Hippocrates called *ponos* (the bit that hurts!), we would be overwhelmed by our hostile environment. Acute disease is actually the process of throwing off unwanted challenges. Usually this is successful. But by untimely interference with the process of resolution – by administering chemical suppression therapy, for example – we are simply driving the toxins or insult underground, where they will emerge later as a more chronic illness.

Homeopathy does the opposite. Far from being a powerful antagonist of disease, it actually mimics and *uses* the disease process to get the cure!

The name homeopathy comes from 'homo-' (same) and 'pathos' (disease, as in pathology). There is a famous Latin maxim: 'Similia Similibus Curentur', which translated means 'Like cures like.' Although the idea has been in use since Hippocrates' time, and the great Paracelsus also wrote comprehensively of it, it fell to German physician Samuel Hahnemann to organize the key principles of homeopathy into a cogent scientific thesis, which he did in his great work *The Organon of Rational Medicine*, published in 1810 (he was 55 at the time).[1]

An example of this so-called 'law of similars' is that substantial doses of deadly nightshade (Belladonna) produce a clinical picture almost identical with scarlet fever (a once-common form of streptococcal tonsillitis which doctors hardly ever see these days). The scarlet fever patient has a, bright red rash (hence the name), burning hot, dry, headachey, maybe even delirious, with wide staring eyes and extreme restlessness. Hahnemann found that if he administered Belladonna to a case of scarlet fever, the results were quite beneficial, sometimes even dramatic.

Potentization

But Hahnemann didn't stop there, and this is where homeopathy indeed seems strange. Hahnemann found that if you *dilute* the active substance, the treatment becomes more effective. The more dilute it is, the more powerful the remedy seems to be. This applies even when the original substance is so dilute there can be no chemical molecules left. Hahnemann called the dilution process *potentization*, since it manifestly made the treatment more powerful.

The apparent illogicality of intensification-by-dilution is what excites so much hostility from conventional doctors. They seem to have a silly fall-back logic which argues: *'It can't work, and therefore it doesn't'*. In fact the results show otherwise. There is an ever-increasing number of scientific trials being published that show homeopathy is an effective and safe alternative to drugs in many conditions. Even so, an editorial in the *Lancet* which accompanied a paper showing that homeopathy worked could not resist sniping with the comment that Hahnemann's theories were 'inherently implausible'.

In fact there is nothing implausible whatever about potentization. It merely requires that one finds the right model. Instead of thinking in terms of the concentration of bio-chemical substances, one has only to think in terms of an information field and realize that this is how homeopathy works. The medicine is carrying a message which knocks out the disease 'similar'. The medicine gets better through dilution, simply because we are diluting out what the technical people call 'noise', meaning the extraneous and unnecessary information which interferes with the message we want carried to the tissues.

But how is this information field conveyed? To understand the mechanism better we have to examine the properties of water, so vital to the life process and bio-energies.

The Peculiar Properties of Water

Every schoolboy and -girl knows that water is a molecule consisting of two hydrogen atoms and one oxygen (H_2O). This molecule has a bi-polar charge – that is, a positive charge at one end and a negative charge at the other. Overall these cancel each other out (making the molecule electrically neutral), but close up this property of electrical polarity has consequences. It means that water molecules can act like tiny magnets, with north and south poles, and 'tag' together in what are known as clusters.

These clumps of molecules are capable of carrying electromagnetic information, rather like signals on magnetic tapes or disks, and it is this peculiar characteristic of water that has immense importance for life energies.

It also has great meaning for therapeutics, because information can be carried to the tissues using the most obvious transporter: the body is made up of almost 70 per cent water. Not only that, but the right sort of energetic information will reach all parts of the whole organism virtually simultaneously.

Unfortunately, but hardly surprisingly, this also means that body systems are susceptible to outside electromagnetic disruption. Nearby electrical fields and even celestial events, such as sun spot activity, can influence the health and dynamics of body tissues. Indeed, popular science author Lyall Watson makes the point in his book *Supernature* that, because of our susceptibility to radiations from space, it is possible to provide a scientific model for the ancient belief system of astrology.[2] We have also seen the rise in the belief that external energy fields, such as high-tension electricity cables, can lead to leukaemia and other unwanted conditions.

To demonstrate the capability of water for retaining information, spectral analyses of homeopathic remedies have been carried out. The resulting graphs of several homeopathic potencies of Belladonna are shown in the figure below. It should be noted that, according to physical science, dilutions of D23 (one-in-ten dilution repeated 23 times) or higher cannot possibly contain any chemical residue. What is measured is an energetic information signal. Even at high dilutions (D30 and D200), frequencies above the positive line are recorded, meaning that *the solution is actually transmitting information.*

This cannot be explained by merely substance-based thinking. There is no 'stuff' or mass present, though in fact it should be explained that school-level physics leads us to consider mass too simplistically. Scientists now recognize 'weighable' matter, which has a rest mass; but also non-weighable matter – one might resort to calling it 'virtual matter' – which has only energetic properties and no detectable rest mass.

Whatever is in the 'solution' or residual water after the chemical has left, it carries recognizable energetic properties. It can interact with the tissues and with the disease process, to effect a cure. It does this by resonance – that is, striking a frequency chord (as in music) where the two oscillators (or notes) together match up and create a much-intensified response.

Your radio set does much the same thing. The incoming signal is very attenuated but when you tune the dial, you are altering a resonator (the amplifier) until it matches; at that point the signal becomes much stronger and can be used in a modulating electrical circuit, without it being drowned out. In other words, the information (broadcast) is singled out from the surrounding 'noise'.

Thus there may be no Belladonna carried by the water, but its 'radio transmission' is still present and will resonate with scarlet fever, or any similar combination of symptoms. In 1988 Professor Jacques Benveniste published a now-famous paper in *Nature* magazine, reporting experiments which showed that extreme dilutions of water solutions of an antibody could still evoke a biological response long after the active substance was diluted away, *provided the solution was agitated after each dilution*.[3] Non-agitated solutions produced little or no effect. This pointed clearly to transmission of information via some kind of water-organizing process. Benveniste was bitterly attacked by his peers and even denounced by Sir John Maddox, the then-editor of *Nature*, who had first commissioned the article. For such an affront on the narrow-minded tenets of science Benveniste lost his government funding and his laboratory was closed down. There were even some attempts to prove he had perpetrated a fraud, but in the end this was toned down to hints that his work was not reproducible by others. Such are the vagaries and fashions of science, as Albert Abrams learned (see Chapter 1).

Classical vs Complex Homeopathy

It is sad to report that controversy has broken out even among homeopathic practitioners. There are two factions: the classic homeopaths, practising in the manner of Hahnemann, and those who use what is known as 'complex homeopathy'. I will briefly address the arguments which seem to be creating the rift so that, in looking at the issues, the reader may learn more about both disciplines.

The major difference is that classical homeopathy argues that there must be only one correct remedy for a patient at any one time. It has to be said that there is no scientific or logical basis for this supposition, merely that 'Hahnemann said so,' but to insist upon it as doctrine risks becoming inflexible and out of step with newer developments. Complex homeopathy on the other hand, as you may suppose from its name, means giving multiple remedies at the same time; or only one remedy, but in a range of several different potencies (called a Homaccord).

But there are more subtle differences in philosophy and method between the two fields.

In general, the complex homeopaths use far lower dilutions, closer to what one might call biological values. Classical homeopathy, on the other hand, hots up at around the 30th centesimal, which means a substance diluted 100-fold repeated 30 times (100^{30}); it can go to MM, meaning diluted 500-fold repeated 500 times (500^{500}). To put this into perspective, from 24C (24th centesimal) onwards the dilutions are so enormous there can be no physical substance left.

Complex homeopaths, on the other hand, are quite happy with mixtures that contain 2X, 3X, 6X, etc., meaning a 10-fold dilution repeated 2, 3 and 6 times respectively. Complex homeopaths also tend to use a great deal more of diluted tissues and disease material, which we might call 'isopathy' though this word has little real impact. What this means is not so much 'treating like with like' as using 'same to heal same' (for example, healthy pig pancreas for pancreatic disease, Tonsilla for tonsillitis, Carcinomium for a lung cancer, and so on). This will be explained more fully below.

Buckshot

The result is that complex homeopathy tends to be less of a one-hit miracle and more of a gradual attrition of the disease process, over a space of several months. Whereas a classical homeopath will stop the remedy the moment it is seen to produce a significant result, a complex homeopath smiles with satisfaction and adds another two months' prescription to the therapy programme.

I bring up this controversy in some detail simply because it strikes at the heart of what we mean (or believe we mean) when we talk about homeopathy as being an 'energy medicine' or based on resonance and information fields.

If we believe our own explanation, then complex homeopathy ought to make the more sense of the two. We are talking about energy signals or information patterns resonating or interacting with sympathetic frequencies in the diseased patient. Therefore if there are a number of frequencies or a 'spread' of energies (like buckshot) at around the right magnitude, there will be more chance of successfully hitting the target. The unwanted resonances, which find no counterpart in the body, should have no interactive effect whatever. They just go away.

Classical homeopathy, one remedy at a time, it is true can produce very impressive results. But if the practitioner is mistaken in the choice of remedy, *or chooses an unsuitable potency*, there may be little or no result. This means added delays and suffering for the patient, while the practitioner tries something new.

There is another simple, all-too-human appeal in complex remedies. If we doctors are honest with ourselves and others, the reality of daily clinical practice reveals that we are far from perfect. With the exception of those individuals with outstanding memories it isn't possible to carry a full working knowledge of all potential remedies. A busy homeopath will often settle for a similar (near enough) rather than a true 'similimum' (exact remedy).

This lack of precision in choosing the similimum results in less effective therapy. Complex remedies are designed, at least in part, to accommodate for this lack of precision.

Complex homeopathy is sometimes called the 'German system', though in view of Hahnemann's nationality one could argue that *both* are the property of that great intellectual and cultured race.

In conclusion, it must be pointed out that all complex homeopaths are flexible enough to use classical remedies in the classical manner when these seem appropriate. We accord great respect to Hahnemann's teachings; but are not restricted needlessly by them.

MESENCHYME THERAPY AND THE MATRIX

In the absence of any objective measurable change at the structural or chemical pathological level, doctors are reluctant to consider 'real' disease and think instead of psychiatric or functional disorder (meaning disordered function of the mind; a euphemism for madness or delusion).

But there is another domain or theatre of disease, which, although ignored by the powerful financial lobby which controls modern medicine, has continued to be researched quietly in Europe and the former Soviet bloc for most of this century. We may term it the 'humoral' nature of disease – that is, disease manifested as a result of disruptive imbalances in the quality and content of the fluid medium in which our organs and cells are suspended. Two central figures in the development of this model, which is also sometimes called Homotoxicology, are the clinician Dr Hans-Heinrich Reckeweg and Professor Alfred Pischinger, the father of modern histochemistry.

The fundamental concept is that of homo- (auto)toxins accumulating in the interstitial (support) fluid and tissues which we call the mesenchyme or 'matrix'.[45] Toxin here does not simply mean pollution or waste matter from cells, but includes the 'memory' of disease and the residues of malfunction and stasis. But I would like to challenge the received wisdom. I suggest that the importance of the biochemistry of these toxins is actually secondary to the deterioration in the ionic energy-conductive properties of the collagen matrix. Remember from Chapter 2 that Georges Lakhovsky predicted that the accumulation of interstitial toxins would cause alterations in electromagnetic oscillation potential, which would alter conductance and resistivity and mean that cells could no longer vibrate at their inherent healthy frequencies.

We shall return to this concept of the intercellular matrix and its variable dielectric status in Chapter 11. For the moment let's just say that what is clear is that there is far more interstitial matter than cells which comprise organs. Thus, in terms of volume alone it makes a great deal of sense to pay attention to this fluid matrix. Yet it is barely mentioned in the medical school curriculum and doctors continue to graduate with no more than a passing knowledge of this vital energetic domain of our bodies.

Far from being what is left when you take away the 'important' structures, the connective tissue matrix is the basic regulation system of the entire organism. Without it the organs could not function in a concerted whole. The matrix is to the organs of the body what the engine, gears and wheels are to the body of a car. A harmonious and well-functioning matrix is synonymous with good health.

This matrix has three obvious functions: nutrition, defence and repair. It carries out these functions in response to a whole gamut of input stimuli, whether energy, hormones, osmotic gradients, electrical impulses, immunological signals, neurotransmitters and, of course, any toxin-irritating presence.

What Reckeweg correctly perceived was that if Pischinger's matrix becomes clouded and sludged up with toxins, then there is a cumulative process of degeneration and decay, leading towards advanced pathological conditions, notably malignancy. The same message as Lakhovsky's. The organism works less and less efficiently until resistance is overcome. Finally the processes of pathology take over and run down the machinery towards death. By the time cancer growths appear, the end may well be close. Reckeweg coined the term 'homotoxicosis' for this sequence.

What homotoxicology does is best thought of as de-polluting the matrix. The skilled use of appropriate complex homeopathic remedies can cleanse or reverse the decay process. It often means using toxin signals, presented homeopathically in the form we call *nosodes*. This drives out the disease process, though unpleasant reactions can appear as the reversal process gets under way. To prevent this we use drainage remedies which speed the elimination of toxins, as described below.

Reckeweg called this cleansing of the matrix and reversal towards a healthy state 'regressive vicariation'. I regard it as a potentially misleading term; I would prefer '*pro*-gressive vicariation', since it gives the idea of improvement. But Reckewcg's chosen expression calls attention to the fact that we are rolling disease backwards, reversing into earlier and better levels of health.

Hering's Law

This reversal of the disease process described by Reckeweg is associated with an older and well-established healing law. It was formulated by the 19th-century American homeopath Constantine Hering, but it applies to many healing disciplines, not just homeopathy. It is a truly great insight into the healing of disease and should be taught in letters of fire to all who aspire to comfort and mend our fellows.

Hering's Law states that, in the course of healing a disease, recovery takes place in three clearly defined ways and that these are signs of meaningful recovery:

1 **Healing is from inside to outside.** Thus a runny nose is an improvement on colitis or asthma. Do *not* diagnose 'rhinitis' and try to prevent the nasal mucus! The response is a healing process and *not* a new diseasc.
2 **Healing is from top to bottom.** Thus a skin rash will clear from the head first and lower limbs last. Keep going!
3 **Healing takes place from the most important organs towards the least important**. Thus irritable bowel could be a sign of therapeutic response from mental illness. You are drawing the disease from the mind into the body.

There is another very important and related aspect to this, which is that during the process of recovery the disease sometimes 'rolls back' through time: symptoms that came last go first; symptoms that preceded those may reappear for a time before they in turn vanish. A child who developed asthma and then migraine may well go temporarily back to asthma when put on an effective remedial programme (this also fits rule 2). It's like putting the mesenchyme 'car' into reverse; you have to go back through all the old familiar landmarks you passed on your way to 'Disease-ville'.

This observation is often tacked onto Hering's Law, though Hering himself did not phrase it so. Reckeweg may not be the first person to recognize the back-track phenomenon, but he was the first to give it a name, albeit the rather clumsy 'regressive vicariation'!

NOSODES

I have hinted that probably the key therapeutic agent of mesenchyme therapy is the *nosode*. A nosode is a homeopathically-prepared sample of disease tissue or biological toxins. These samples are negative energy signals of substances which hurt or poison the body, or dangerous tissue. For example Carcinomium, made from cancer tissue, is very hostile to the body, as you would expect. Any disease-producing virus, bacteria or parasite would automatically make a nosode; Dr Edward Bach, famous for his flower remedies discussed shortly, actually made some of the first-ever bacterial nosodes by potentizing vaccines, still known as the Seven Bach Nosodes.[6] Modern advances in the field of EAV and beyond have made it quite clear that pesticides, heavy metal poisons, electro-pathic stress, medicines and numerous other stressors all have the essential character of nosodes.

Nosodes are potentially strong remedies and may provoke an illness in response to their administration. Even though the measles or TB may not be present, except as a virtual signal, the body still reacts as if the disease was in progress. The tissues fight back. The patient feels bad once again; we call this a 'healing crisis'.

Drainage Remedies

Notwithstanding Hering's law, we solve this problem with the use of what are known as 'drainage remedies'. As the name implies, drainage remedies are substances which can provoke speedier toxin removal, whether by stimulating the kidneys, liver or other excretion pathway (diarrhoea is seen by holistic practitioners as nothing more than toxin-flushing and often comes on in response to a treatment). We can categorize drainage according to organ: pancreas, liver, gut, etc. Or we can grade it according to power: mild, gentle, medium, forte and 'ultra' preparations.

It is said that almost any pathological or nosode preparation is capable of working as a drainage remedy, if the dilution is right. This will happen if it is not too forceful (lower potencies) and does not provoke more quickly than it cleanses. One of my patients joked about 'taking her diseases in water'!

It might seem tempting to administer the strongest drainage remedy possible, to give a good flushing to the system. But that is to think like a drug-prescribing physician. All energy medicine is conceptualized on the principle of the so-called 'minimum dose'.

What does this mean?

Adey's Window and Arndt-Schulz's Law

Elementary-school science drums into us the linear or quadratic relationship and we are taught that if a quantity of some substance has a particular effect, then larger amounts will perforce induce a greater effect. But this is often not so.

There are very good biological reasons for the magic of the minimum. If the body is subjected to too strong an input signal, this often has a negative rather than a positive effect. This can be likened to turning up a radio set so loud that it begins to distort. The extra volume is counter-productive and the programme broadcast will be heard better by turning down the volume to a more comfortable level. Overdosing is the way in which many drugs work. I am convinced that much allopathic medicine is simply poisoning out some part of our physiology; for example, painkillers poison the full working of the nervous system.

Virtual Medicine practitioners have come to understand that

the biological information field is paramount, and that the field only needs to be modulated slightly for there to be a major change in output. This is summed up in another holistic principle known as Arndt-Schulz's Law, which applies to homeopathic prescribing but again also to many other interacting living systems:

- A small stimulus will provoke positively
- A larger signal has no further effect
- A very large signal actually has a suppression effect.

W. Ross Adey of Loma Linda University showed this effect experimentally while studying calcium influx in irradiated animal brain cells. He showed that the brain cells not only responded to quite specific frequencies (approx 10 Hz), but did so only at extremely low intensities.[7]

There was, in effect, only a very tiny spread of values in which the optimum effect could be detected. Outside that range either nothing happened, or function was suppressed. This gives us a new term, the *Adey Window*, meaning an effective low-level band or response-slot. Adey received the Hans Selye Award for this holistic insight in March 1999, at Montreux in Switzerland.

Hormesis

This is a good point to bring in the little-known phenomenon of *hormesis*. Numerous studies have shown that minute doses of poisons have a stimulating, tonic and anti-toxic effect. Strychnine, for example, appeared empirically in many medical 'tonics' in former times. In experiments carried out at the University of Wyoming, minimal exposures to potentially lethal radiation actually extended the lives of insects, rabbits and other creatures. It seems that heavy metals and even antibiotics can have the same effect in small enough quantities.

This propensity for toxins to be beneficial when below the threshold level we call 'hormesis'. Hormesis stimulates the cellular defence systems.

There is the possibility of two separate lifespans – the one we are familiar with in principle, which is the maintenance of home-ostatic balance as described by Claude Bernard in the 19th century, and the other caused by tipping the balance slightly unfavourably against the organism, so that the body is forced to make self-preserving changes. This can be called the 'stress-induced lifespan'.

Researchers Patricia Neafsey at Tufts University School of Medicine and Harold Oxenbaum at Merill Dow Research Institute have reviewed the evidence pointing to this phenomenon and concluded: 'Assessment of mortality data from modern bioassay studies indicate that low dose animal exposure to a variety of toxic agents can ... through an unknown mechanism, promote health and prolong life-longevity hormesis.'[8]

These conclusions are thought-provoking, and the relevance for humans is yet to be established. But clearly here is a version of the Arndt-Schulz principle and yet further evidence for the benefits of nosode therapy.

Specificity

It is important to note that nosodes are not necessarily given only for the disease to which they relate (for example giving a 'flu nosode in a case of 'flu). In fact that is to underestimate and miss the importance and applicability of this new therapeutic range. Empirically it has been found by Voll, Schimmel and others, that certain diseases associate with particular nosodes. Conversely, some nosodes come up time and again as trouble-makers in many different conditions. Childhood vaccines are particularly notorious in this respect. I think we can go some way towards answering the mystery about where the present post-war epidemic of allergies has come from. At least part of the reason is the child-hood vaccination programme, dropping toxins on the immune system, spleen, etc., which then results in malfunction. The child may avoid the whooping cough or diphtheria, only to suffer with many more obscure and difficult-to-treat symptoms later in life.

I myself prefer to use homeopathic 'vaccination' in which the body is accustomed to the noxious agent, along the lines of hormesis. It is safer, painless, cheaper and does not have the same side-effects as true vaccination. (Lest you fear it won't work, it is interesting to note that in the last great diphtheria epidemic in Glasgow, just before the advent of antibiotics, over 50 per cent of the children died with conventional therapy, yet not one fatality occurred at the city's homeopathic hospital).[9]

Here are some examples of the diversity of effects of nosodes, though the full reference range of many hundreds of items is a matter of considerable learning and remains the intellectual property of a well-trained practitioner.

Disease Condition	Nosode Indication
acne	tuberculinum, bacillinum, psorinum
arthritis	streptococcinum, staphylococcinum, apis mellifica, variolinum, vaccinium, influenzinum
breast cancer	tuberculinum, medorrhinum, carcinosin, syphilinum, variolinum
diabetes	parotidinum, diphtherinum, tuberculinum, bacillinum
migraine	diphtherinum, variolinum, vaccinium
prostatitis	tuberculinum, diphtherinum, pertussin
sciatica	influenzinum, staphylococcinum, streptococcinum
warts	medorrhinum

One can reverse the starting place and view each nosode as a *polyvalent* remedy – that is, capable of reaching out and de-energizing many different disease conditions. Thus:

Nosode	Useful in Treating
Herpes (all)	arthritis, canker sores, spleen, shingles, heart, nerve, pancreas
Morbillinum	hypertension, multiple sclerosis, neurological disorders
Syphilinum	swollen knees (especially in women), brain cancer, heart valve disorders, prostatitis, chronic gynaecological problems
Typhoidinum	intestinal complaints, liver, gall bladder, spleen, heart
Varicellinum	arthritis, myocardial disease, multiple sclerosis, cranial nerve palsies, shingles

MIASM

A miasm is one of the most powerful influences in health and disease I know, yet the least acknowledged or understood. The word was introduced by Hahnemann, but I prefer to think of it as a 'genetic toxin', since this term gives a far clearer idea of what we think we are dealing with. Basically a miasm means a shadow or disease 'imprint' which is inherited down the generations.

All observant doctors are aware that disease and disturbance tend to run in families, and can be likened to a kind of family blight. This is not to mean a specific replicated genetic disorder carried by the genes such as, for example, haemophilia or Freidrich's ataxia. The sickliness can manifest itself in many different ways, each individual suffering differently from the others in his or her family tree but all bound by the commonality of being a somewhat weakened or unhealthy bunch.

This idea may seem to be an attempt to revive Lamarck's discredited theory of evolution, which said that an organism's responses to environmental stressors could be passed on to offspring. This is now held not to be true; the Darwinian/Mendelian dogma reigns, which states that only the factors carried in the genes can be inherited. Rigidity of this degree sounds suspiciously like yet another road-block in scientific thinking; a fashion that will one day have to be exposed to common sense and revised.

To Hahnemann a miasm was something more in the nature of a primitive illness, a throwback. He named three in particular: Syphilis (or Luesinum), Sycosis, and Psora. Briefly, syphilis has ulcerating tendencies; sycosis (meaning from gonorrhoea) is congestive, leading to deposits and tumour formation; while psora is a protean disturbance which relates to functional imbalances of all kinds. Psora is said to have formed in the time of the Plague (the Black Death).

Antoine Nebel and Henry C Allen added Tuberculinum, which many practitioners now regard as the pre-eminent miasm, presumably since it is but one generation removed from today's population stock.[10] Among the fall-out diseases from this inherited toxin one can list asthma, eczema, hay fever, food allergies, chronic sinusitis, migraines, mental illness of various kinds including retardation and subnormality, irritable bowel, colitis, heart trouble, diabetes, Hodgkin's disease and even leukaemia.

Leon Vannier added a fifth, which is the Oncotic (cancer) miasm. It is characterized by changes in body odour, warts, excrescences, sores that refuse to heal and a sallow skin, somewhat like that of malignant cachexia.

It is also fashionable to consider the emergence of at least two new miasms: Candida and Chemical Sensitivity; Sugar Glut may very likely become a third modern miasm. I suggest we call the Candida miasm, if we can agree there is one, 'Mouldy'. I introduced the term 'mouldy patient' in my book *The Allergy Handbook*[11] and it seems to me a far bigger issue than just Candida; the patient becomes sensitized to a wide variety of moulds and yeasts. Unquestionably it is brought about by overuse of antibiotics, made worse by our obsession for refined carbohydrate and sugar, which results in a great deal of unnatural fermentable matter in the gut.

May we say then what a miasm is? I think in the light of modern understanding of energetic medicine it is possible to go beyond Hahnemann's hypothesis and say we are surely dealing with some kind of transmittable information field with its accompanying energetic disturbance. It appears 'etheric' or non-material in quality, but that is because hitherto we have not had the electronic means to search in the outer energy shell, except by dowsing. The fact is, miasms show up repeatedly on comprehensive testing of the electro-dermal screening (EDS) sort (see Chapter 8). We know they are there. Treatment consists of giving the homeopathic similar most exactly pertaining to the shadow. EAV and remedy testing can help us to identify and treat miasms with greater accuracy than ever before.

Casebook: Male, 10 Years

From the age of three the patient suffered from repeated vexatious sore throats and ear trouble. He fell steadily behind other children his age in scholastic performance. His tonsils and adenoids had been removed (no improvement) and finally his parents were told by an ear nose and throat (ENT) surgeon that the trouble was caused by allergies and the boy would suffer from this all his life.

Analysis showed that the predominant stressor was TB miasm and an acquired measles toxin. The indicated miasm and nosode were started and continued at appropriate repeat intervals over several months.

The ear and throat condition cleared up rapidly and has never reappeared. The boy's mental and physical slowness, which had been such a worry to his parents and teachers, soon abated and he was able to hold his own with his peers.

BACH FLOWER REMEDIES

One cannot consider energy medicine, particularly the information-in-water-alcohol kind, without giving some consideration to Bach's flower remedies. These are superb information medicines of the virtual sort and a great gift to the healer from a humanistic but strange man.

Despite the Germanic sounding name, Bach (pronounced like batch) was actually of Welsh origin, born near Birmingham in 1886. He practised homeopathy in fashionable Harley Street in the 1920s. After 1930 he gave up his successful practice to study plants and trees and their psychological effects, culminating in the publication of the book *The Twelve Healers and Other*

Remedies.[12] Today there are 38 remedies in all, ranging from gentian, through wild oat, to oak.

One outstanding remedy called 'Rescue Remedy' (a mixture of Cherry Plum, Clematis, Impatiens, Rock Rose and Star of Bethlehem) seems to have a special place. I have seen it effective against shock, trauma, children's hysteria, travel sickness, rashes and even bees refusing to pollinate. It is one of medicine's truly *great* remedies and should be in the emergency cupboard in every home. A word of caution, however: it is a shock remedy and if you take it when not in shock it can predispose unpleasant shock-like reactions. Never use Rescue Remedy prophylactically (as a preventative).

Bach was what is sometimes called a 'sensitive' – that is, a person who has the gift for unusual psychic perceptions. I have noticed that surprisingly many of these people, for all their gifts, are not very healthy. Bach was no exception and died tragically young. Maybe their gifts are the *result* of being out of focus with the rest of us. I have seen this effect so often in my allergy patients; I soon became aware that feeling unreal and depersonalized has a certain transcendent aspect.

What Bach came to investigate was the way in which psychological attitudes prevented the normal healing and recovery process. It is usually forgotten today, when his remedies are in fashion for every kind of psychological hang-up, that what he originally proposed to treat were merely the barriers to healing.

He carried out his investigations by touching plants or the dew which settled on flowers and noting the emotional feeling it gave to him. He collected the coded botanical information by shining sunlight through the petals onto a brandy and water stock (sunlight method); or by boiling down the plant to create a concentrated extract or tincture (boiling method). Only one remedy, Rock Water, is not botanical in origin but is exactly what its name suggests and comes from mountain streams.

Bach remedies are unquestionably bio-informational in character, which is why they are reviewed here. They work mainly at the etheric or trans-dimensional level, and are in every sense a 'virtual remedy'. A person sometimes has only to touch or hold the bottle to get an emotional release. Your author actually burst into tears on picking up a book describing these remedies; I tell this only because I think it says more about the remedies than about me! Make of this strange occurrence what you will.

One theoretical objection might be the concern that what applied to Bach and his other-wordly persona would not necessarily apply to the rest of us, or at least not in the same manner. However, this hypothetical problem has largely been taken care of with the passage of time; the remedies today enjoy enormous popularity, and world-wide sales attest to their astonishing efficacy.

Clinical Applications

I can only echo Bach's original view and say that, in my own electronic diagnosis and therapy system called the Acupro (see Chapter 8), I find I sometimes need to add one or more flower essences to the treatment tanks before the Indicator Drop will vanish and we know that the therapy programme will succeed. It is axiomatic that much disease has a psychological element and that unless this is addressed, even by something as gentle as a coded flower message, the patient may have limited recovery.

Casebook: Female, 37 years

Dr Sam Williams tells a remarkable story of a woman patient who had been severely traumatized by a road traffic accident several years before. The emotional impact was, to say the least, unnerving. Ever since, she had been unable to leave her home without being wrapped in heavy blankets against traffic noise and blindfolded, so that she could not see anything connected with cars or roads.

In this pathetic state she was driven to his office and unwrapped, looking very miserable and dishevelled. His Acupro system sang out the flower remedies, including Mimosa, which is 'fear of known things' and the patient went home with her formula, unconvinced.

Despite two decades of EAV experience, no-one was more surprised than Sam when, next morning, the woman drove herself to his office alone, dressed to the nines, and handed him the bottle back in person, saying 'I don't think I need these any more Doc, but thanks!'

She was on her way to her first shopping spree.

In conclusion, Bach has given rise to a whole culture based on flower essences. At least two additional schools have emerged, one in Australia using Pacific Flower Remedies, and the other from the West Coast of the US, the so-called California Essences. Notable is the Flower Essence Society founded in 1979 by Richard Katz. Doubtless there will be more and more expansion as other adepts add their own contributions.

IMPRINTING

This review of the main available remedy modalities for EDS and Virtual Medicine practitioners would be incomplete without describing a sort of trade secret called 'imprinting'.

Dr Franz Morell, the MO- of MORA (Chapter 6), discovered that sometimes during the course of BER medicine, the patient would actually recover if the remedy was 'played back', like a recording, into the patient's tissues, either through the bar electrode or directly via the acupuncture point through which the necessary data was accessed. Very occasionally just being exposed briefly to the remedy while it was being tested was sufficient to produce a therapeutic result. Although the benefit could sometimes last a considerable time, these responses were usually of short duration, often disappearing as soon as the remedy signal was removed from the circuit and the point retested. But Morell discovered in his experiments that if the chosen remedy oscillation was amplified 8–10 times and then played back, the result could last for weeks, months or even indefinitely.[13]

This is basically what the MORA machine does. The rest of us, who don't use one, have to adopt some other means of attaining the same result. This leads almost naturally to the idea of *imprinted* medicines, which can extend the electronically-derived treatment process once the patient has gone home.

An imprinted medicine is one in which the supposed

therapeutic electromagnetic message, derived from the Acupro library or similar sources, or a real sample on the input honey-comb, is transferred into a mixture of water and brandy. In other words, instead of giving the patient Echinacea, we play the information signature of Echinacea into the remedy bottle and give the patient that instead.

Lest you think the whole idea absurd, let me tell you that many of the cases reviewed in this book were treated in this way. The very dramatic story of Ed Butler of the Platters (page 140) was treated with only imprinted remedies, since I carry no nosodes of 'flu virus. The machine detected the disease and told me what would eliminate it.

We talk about the individual 'vibrational signature' of substances, herbs, homeopathics, enzymes and other beneficial substances. It ought to be quite logical and indeed scientific, if we really are dealing with nothing other than energy signals, to be able to transfer the energetic signal to a carrier fluid or other medium. I have already explained that the peculiar properties of water and brandy mean that these are especially suited to carrying transferred electromagnetic signals.

We can call this electro-homeopathy.

CAUTION

In view of what has just been stated, it would be remiss of me not to point out a potential danger. If we can imprint the 'signature' of a substance in liquid, it follows that the same would apply even regarding unfriendly or toxic material. Many years ago at an advanced think tank, I heard a proposal that boiling water in an electric kettle or using electric heating rings to cook our food might impart what we ate or drank with hostile electromagnetic energies (bear in the mind that mains frequency of around 50–60 Hz is particularly damaging to biological systems).

I am sorry to say that I somewhat scorned this possibility at the time (1982). At least I should have kept an open mind. Almost two decades on I have learned enough to know that this is more than a theoretical possibility. We certainly *do* imprint liquids with unintended energy codes. A beer on the top of the

TV may have a little of your favourite (or most hated) programme in it! The question which remains unanswered is, can imbibing these imprinted substances have detrimental effects on health?.

I have no idea of the answer. But I would say this: keep all medicines and remedies, even vitamins and minerals, *well away* from any source of electromagnetic radiation, such as computers, TVs and microwaves. Otherwise they will almost certainly be spoiled.

THAT MAN BENVENISTE AGAIN

I have already referred in this chapter to the way in which Jacques Benveniste caused a scandal when he published proof of what came to be known as 'the memory of water' in the scientific journal *Nature*. Now he is back with even more radical theories about the energetic signatures of molecules.

Benveniste's more recent work suggests that it will be possible to record electronically the specific characteristics of a remedy or any other substance, such as adrenalin, nicotine and caffeine, or the immunological pattern of viruses or other pathogens. These recordings can subsequently be played back and even transmitted through telephone cables and thus on to the Internet. I find it a sad irony that Albert Abrams already did this, in effect, in 1924. But his brilliance has been somehow forgotten as his star fell.

Biological systems, Benveniste then goes on to assert, can be activated far away from the triggering molecules, simply by playing back the electronic signature of the substance in question. Even more improbably, we may be able to 'hear' these signals acoustically in time. All molecules are made up of atoms, which are constantly vibrating and emitting infra-red radiation. These infra-red vibrations have been recognized for years and are known to be highly specific to each atom or substance. Their resonance frequencies actually fall in the range which is audible to the human ear (20 to 20,000 Hz) and it is this low-frequency pattern which Benveniste records and uses to transmit the molecular characteristics. He claims to have sent caffeine and curare signals across the Atlantic by ordinary telecommunications from a laboratory in Europe to another in the US and obtained a measurable effect at the other end. If this is true, one science columnist wrote, it will undoubtedly earn Benveniste a Nobel Prize.[14]

So far, Benveniste reports that he can only record and play back a message. He and his team cannot yet recognize patterns or identify unknown substances from their recording.

One exciting aspect of his hypothesis is that it explains the manner in which many remedies or physiological substances have an almost instantaneous effect throughout the organism. This can be much too fast to be explained by humoral or bio-chemical means. The usual proposed mechanism is a neurologi-cal one. But Benveniste's model makes more sense. It also sheds light on the phenomenon of specific biological receptors. The usual explanation is one of a 'lock and key' mechanism; that is, the receptor site has a physical shape which admits only the cor-rect trigger molecule. I have always viewed this as specious and remarked earlier in the book that allergic reactions, or *recoveries due to therapy*, can be so instantaneous as to beggar the normal pathways. Benveniste's proposal of transmitting molecules and 'tuned' receptor sites (like a radio aerial) fits these clinical obser-vations far better. In his view, it would take only a tiny alteration of the receptor to de-tune it, so that it no longer responds.

I am grateful to Benveniste for progress with understanding one of the last major building blocks of the Virtual Medicine par-adigm. I would also remind the reader of Roger Coghill's com-ments on DNA and other cell molecules 'transmitting' the body's genetic message, resulting in species-specific growth (page 21).

CHAPTER 8

ELECTRO-DERMAL
COMPUTER SCREENING

We now come to the moment when the promise of this book's title is close to fulfilment. Picture the scene in a 21st-century doctor's surgery. After the preliminaries, the patient sits down in front of a computer display, picks up the passive electrode and the doctor begins to touch the patient's skin at certain of Voll's electro-acupuncture points which we call the central measurement points (CMPs), one on each vessel or meridian. The sensor is similar to the Dermatron but is now hitched to a high-powered desktop PC and the two talk to each other electronically. There is a picture of a hand skeleton; a bright red dot wanders across each digit, beep-beep-beep. After every measurement the

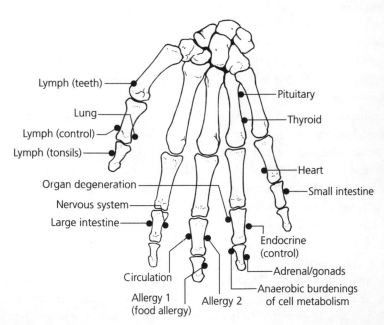

doctor clicks a button and the reading goes into the computer's memory to be stored. We now have an electronic file which can be called up any time in the future and printed out for study or even for the patient to take home a personal copy. Times have changed!

Some things are the same, however. This is still electro-acupuncture according to Voll (EAV): there are two meridians to each finger digit and two to each toe, making a total of 40 readings in all. But when this preliminary stage is complete, by pressing a key the doctor brings up on the screen an attractive coloured graph. It shows all the CMP measurement values; right and left sides are in different colours for ease of identification; Indicator Drops (IDs) are marked as white bands and stand out clearly.

The doctor pauses and looks deep in thought for a few moments. He taps the white marks on the screen and announces: 'Your spleen meridian is down, the endocrine's not so good and something is disturbing the large intestine. The liver is high, which means it is having to detox hard; but there is no drop so no liver damage so far.' He then presses a couple of keys and goes into 'branching', which means that he now studies the spleen meridian in more detail, passing along it point by point, recording all the values and IDs.

You are watching what it says on the screen out of the corner of your eye: lymphocyte function of the upper body – click; serous coating of the spleen (what's that, for goodness sake?) – click; lymphocyte function of the lower body – click; erythrocyte function (that's the red blood cells) – click; reticulo-endothelial system ... the what? You decide this is all very high tech. But the doctor touches a spot just above your left ankle – click, and announces he has finished that step.

Once again, due to the power of the computer, he taps in a key-code and the sequence of measurements is displayed for review as a table showing highs and lows and the size of the Indicator Drops. The 12-point ID which was found on the CMP reappears on SP2, the reference point for 'lower body leukocyte function'. The doctor is satisfied that this is probably what was disturbing the spleen meridian. Something in the lower body is producing an energetic disturbance that upsets or overstresses the lymphocyte function down there. This could cause a chain reaction, since we need our lymphocytes for defence.

Really upset lymphocytes could even mean leukaemia. There is a problem. But what?

DATABASE

Next, as I think of it, comes *Dr Kildare Meets Chinese Traditional Medicine in Cyberspace*. The doctor calls up a comprehensive database of disease entities and possible cures. On my own system there are over 25,000 entries. This is fairly typical for software packages of this type.

By highlighting an entry and pressing the return key, the doctor can access the energy signal named there on the screen. He can then compare it with what is coming from the disease zone; he does this by touching Spleen 2 with the probe, where he found the biggest drop. He no longer looks for IDs but is probing to see if there is a resonance. This is shown by a reading at or very close to Voll's balanced reading of 50. This means a 'yes' from the body.

But the doctor still has to make choices: could it be a virus? A parasite? Malaria maybe; that's likely for spleen for anyone who has been to the tropics ... and so on. But he can check his theories very quickly and begin to establish the likely cause of the trouble.

The software programmer, if he is good, will already have programmed in some suggestions which relate to that meridian. For the spleen one would give high priority to testing infectious mononeucleosis, 'flu, Tuberculinum, Diphtherinum, pertussis, tetanus, malaria, Variolinum (smallpox) and hepatitis A, B and C. These would accordingly come at the top of the list.

Gall-bladder would give a different range of suggestions. On my system the first 10 offers (in order) are: cholelithiasis (gallstone), amoeba, streptococcus, staphylococcus, 'flu, Diphtherinum, Variolinum, TB and hepatitis A and B.

The nerve-degeneration channel would put measles and rubella in the first 10; also probably Syphilinum and Medorrhinum (gonorrhoea code), which may be less obvious.

This is a good moment to reiterate that EAV gives one a completely different perspective on the origins and nature of disease. Remember that we are testing an energetic signal. This is not looking for antibodies to the micro-organism or a sample culture to 'prove' that this is what the patient has *right now*. Indeed, it generally turns out to be something *from long ago*. Time and again, when we question the patient, he or she can remember the problem that the machine has unearthed and says is still causing trouble. Sometimes the patient will telephone next day, excited, to say that a parent or some other relative confirms the diagnosis which the patient was unable to remember personally at the screening session. Childhood diseases and vaccinations come up over and over again as underpinning disease in later life. The energy disturbance is still around, provoking trouble years later. The proof of such a contentious remark, of course, is that when you lift the signal, the patient begins to improve!

More of this later.

THE PRODUCT LIBRARY

We can think in terms of a 'library' of signals available to the practitioner to check against. Among the likely categories found in a computer database for this sort of testing are signals of:

- alcohol products
- amino acids
- ayurvedic herbs
- bacteria nosodes
- chemicals
- biological age
- geopathic stress
- colour therapies
- chakras
- dental materials
- enzymes
- flower remedies
- herbal remedies
- gems and crystals
- hormones
- environmentals
- essential oils
- food allergies
- grass pollens
- habit drugs

- heavy metals
- homeopathics: combinations, drainage, singles
- polychrests *(a subdivision of homeopathics, polychrests are major remedies with great impact and many ramifications)*
- miasms
- minerals
- parasites
- pesticides
- phenolics
- pollens
- sarcodes *(healthy tissue signals used as support)*
- Scheussler tissue salts
- tree pollens
- vaccines
- venoms
- viruses
- vitamins

At first such a huge database can seem very overwhelming, there are so many choices; how is it possible for one brain to take it all in? Actually, it isn't too daunting.

First, it has to be said that no one individual does or possibly could use and come to grips with *all* of it; I mean understand all the possibilities to a professional level. There have to be selections and generally we work to our strengths. My system has chakras listed: I've never even opened this section for a patient, since in all honesty I wouldn't know what to do with a chakra that was out of balance. But I understand nosodes, such as bacteria, viruses, parasites, chemical toxins, vaccines and allopathic drugs, and I 'find' these a great deal, since I am looking for them. As with all EAV systems, allergies and nutritional guidance is a strong point.

The second vital point which brings it within human capability is that computers by their very nature can help a lot when searching, namely breaking things down relentlessly with either-or logic. It is possible to test a hundred possibilities, then halve it and test that, then halve again, and so on. There is a mathematical principle that you can get down to one item with just six, or at the most seven, decisions using this split logic. Thus if there is a single item you want buried somewhere in a hundred possibilities, it can take less than 20 seconds to find it; such is the power of computers.

The really *great* thing about these computer programmes is that they will tell you first: *'Yes there is something in this list of test substances'*. You don't have to waste time searching fruitlessly in sub-folders that are not relevant to the case.

A refinement which is added to the LISTEN system – one of the first such software packages; the name stands for Life Information Systems Ten, and was developed by James Hoyte Clark of Orem, Utah – is that the search is made 'blind': the items on the list are kept hidden from the practitioner until after he has decided which agent is the real culprit or the desired remedy. This eliminates any prejudgement by the practitioner, which can bedevil objective results and is a good answer to criticism that EAV is really just sophisticated 'dowsing'.

However, it needs to be said that in these advanced systems, nothing can take the place of clinical experience on the part of the practitioner. The machine does not (yet) think for us. It does not 'know', for example, that a large bowel ID, with intestinal lymphatic stress and toxic liver burdenings, would suggest a parasite high in the probable list, or that a head focus is likely to be tonsils, teeth and then sinuses, in that order.

ELECTRO-DERMAL SCREENING

We call this investigative process with computer-based Voll technology electro-dermal screening (EDS). With necessary caution, I can state that it holds great promise for the future. Considering that we are merely in the first decade or two of its development, it already surpasses expectation. As more is learned and scientific studies using this approach give us even more insight and understanding into what is happening in disease, then I think we may soon see a time when it is the basis of any sensible medical practice. EDS is a quick, non-invasive and painless method of health screening.

There are a number of systems you might run into, all much of a muchness. I do not wish to become involved in arguing the relative merits of each; cost, software facilities and back-up service would all be part of such an evaluation. But of the ones I have heard of, I can suggest good results from the following: The BEST (bio-energetic stress test) system, LISTEN, Acupro, Avatar, Clinic-in-a-Case and Biomed. Now the MORA firm have put together a machine which has a computer library and could, fairly, be said to have joined this group of devices. Since it also combines the facility of bioresonance (see Chapter 6) with EAV and a database, it is perhaps the best machine on the market at this time.

For medico-legal reasons, in the US these devices are considered a 'new device' to be used for investigational purposes only. This is a good description. But actually I have found them also educational. One does learn about illness in a totally new way by exploring each case for the consequences which finally led to the onset of disease.

The really critical factor in getting results is not the software but the operator's ability. The most sophisticated device in the world is less than useful if not backed up by the knowledge and skill requisite for using it. It is still fundamentally EAV and is subject to all the difficulties in objectivity found with this approach. We have to be honest and recognize the drawbacks, as well as the strengths.

Tanks

There are many advantages to using a computer, not the least of which is what we call 'the holding tanks'. These can store diagnostic information and useful remedies and return the signal of their contents to the site being skin-tested. My system has eight holding tanks in all. Remedies can be directed into any one of the eight and stored there, to be played back and tested against the tissue, in company with later choices.

These tanks can be switched in and out, which gives us a number of potential refinements. Thus we sometimes see that a remedy is effective on a particular meridian but when later treatments, especially nosodes or stressors are introduced for treating other organs, that the first point becomes unsettled. We can switch tanks or substances in or out until we find which is the culprit. We can test the whole planned treatment regimen against several points consecutively.

A tank behaves just like a honeycomb on the Dermatron or

Vega machine. Filters can be put into the tanks and held there for subsequent testing. They also allow us to organize our thinking a little: I prefer to put my flower remedies in one tank, allergy results in another, homeopathics in a third, biological age in a fourth, and so on.

Most systems will allow one to imprint individual tanks to make individualized remedies.

Filters

A wise EDS specialist will take a leaf out of Schimmel's book and call up the Vega filters for tolerance (Ferrum metallicum D800), compatibility (Manganum metallicum D26) and effectiveness (Ferrum metallicum D26). These can be put into tank 1 and remain there as a background filtering process. This ensures that any remedies chosen are likely to be not only effective but well tolerated by the patient and compatible with other aspects of therapy.

Once a reading-stressed area is found, then a remedy programme needs to be found which will relieve the problem. Obviously an effective remedy must be able to eliminate the ID. We are, in effect, interviewing the body's cells and asking the tissues what they want. Operator knowledge is important, but with such a vast database on tap what he knows becomes less of an issue.

At first the budding EDS practitioner will tend to go along with nosodes and other suggestions put forward by the software. But gradually the practitioner learns his or her own path through this database.

As a comment, I have started to use Bach's flower remedies simply because, on many occasions, I could not get rid of the ID until I included these; often more than one at a time, which will incense the purists. The inference is, of course, that all disease has some psychological component. Unless that is addressed there is resistance to treatment, as Bach postulated. Time and again the patient will recognize themselves in the description of the flower remedy or, if not, a close relative will speak for them and confirm how uncannily accurate EDS can be.

A typical EDS machine is capable of potentizing energy

signals. Thus if Candida albicans is a reading pathogen, as part of its software capability the machine is able to offer for testing a Candida 4X, 6X, 8X, 12X, 24X and so on. The centesimal scale is also represented (see Chapter 7). Generally these are 'softer' in nature. They are more applicable to chronic or constitutional conditions. My system, the Acupro, even allows testing of a range of 5X potencies, which can be used in correlation with the allergy testing and neutralization system known as Miller's method.[1]

Thus the practitioner can make up his or her own remedy formulas by combining different strengths of different substances (which can be imprinted, as described on page 128). Also supplied are what we call *accompanying remedies*, which are selected for each organ concerned. These give lift and support for the organ and help to eliminate toxins. They are in fact specially chosen drainage remedies (see page 119).

Many proprietary remedy brands are included with these machines, such as Heel products, Reckeweg, Pascoe and Futureplex, to name a few. Again, practitioners tend to develop prescribing favourites, but it often happens that only one remedy reads 'OK' and this is what the body is saying it really wants, regardless of preferences.

Accuracy

Most EDS systems take advantage of the computer modality to allow the practitioner to set a definition of 'yes' or 'no' when choosing a remedy. Voll's classic 50 is a theoretical mean. Some practitioners will take anything between 45 and 55 as a positive acceptance by the tissues. I prefer to tune mine at 48 – 52, but since the Acupro takes anything borderline as a 'yes' this degree of accuracy can be very inconvenient at times.

The difficult part is getting the probe pressure just right. Too much or too little pressure will markedly alter the reading. I would say that the touch required is every bit as fine as getting a correct note on a violin string. The Avatar claims to have the advantage that a feather touch is what the system is set up to operate on. This is supposed to be more reproducible, though I do not know on what premise.

Casebook: Male, 57 Years

I was called to see Ed Butler of the Platters singing group. He had just had a massive right-sided stroke, a few days after completing his last recording session. He was now severely incapacitated and sitting disconsolately in a wheelchair. EDS screening showed a major drop on the nervous channel, which was hardly surprising. But what surprised me was that the read was on the *right*. Yet, as everyone knows, the motor nerves cross over before leaving the cranium and the left brain controls the right-sided musculature.

Notwithstanding, I chose to believe what the machine was telling me. I used the right-side as a reference zone. A search for pathogens revealed a loud and unmistakable signal for 1975 'flu. I checked with Ed who, even though it was 23 years previously, remembered clearly having a bad attack and being confined to bed for two weeks. 'That was the start of your stroke,' I told him. In my earlier *Allergy Handbook* I have already pointed out the great potential of 'flu virus to cause considerable neurological damage.

I made up some X-potencies of this pathogen and offered it to the Voll point; it showed a big improvement but the reading was still dropping to a degree. I added some gentle drainage and homeopathic Co-enzyme compositum (a Heel product), to reinvigorate the metabolic process. The read had almost disappeared. Finally, I decided to try flower remedies; including one or two of these did the trick. I gave Ed the remedy the machine had selected for him. In the meantime he was having energetic healing of the 'hands of light' type.

The very next day I had a call that he could move his thumb. Only six weeks into a massive cerebro-vascular accident this was indeed startling. Good recoveries are possible, but we think in terms of 12 – 18 months, not just a few weeks. In any case this was less than 24 hours after starting the 'virtual' remedy.

Over the next few weeks he improved steadily but then pegged. At this point I recognized the remedy was exhausted due to the heat of our Spanish summer, because it had begun to happen with several other patients. I refreshed his remedy, taking the chance to add a couple of items suggested by the repeat test. Once again, the *next day*, I had a call that he was now able to stand on his legs, provided he kept his weight off the weak side. He soon learned to walk and within six months he was back singing in public; an altogether remarkable recovery from a potentially disastrous episode.

I give due credit to the energetic healers, but the immediate response to the remedy indicated by the Acupro is unarguable. Ed's grit and determination were also, of course, major factors.

OTHER REMEDIES

Yet another advantage of the flexible complex homeopathy approach emerges in the EDS domain. It is possible to give 'remedies' of a non-disease modality. For example, we can intervene in metabolic pathways by giving potentized enzyme similimums. Often I find that a person is loaded with toxins and quite sick, with low personal and metabolic energies. It takes quite a lot of internal cellular energy to push out toxins, maybe against a chemical gradient. Thus a vicious circle is established. It may require the use of enzymes of the Kreb's cycle to bring metabolism back up to speed, before the patient can recover. Mixtures such as Heel's 'Co-enzyme compositum' can really help any detox programme by stimulating chemical energy pathways. The patient usually reports subjective increases in energy levels.

We can also administer homeopathically-potentized support signals of substances like essential fatty acids (GLA and EPA), vitamins or minerals. This is not the same as supplementation, which I would always give 'in the physical' as we say. But often the process of uptake and utilization of such nutrient substances is enhanced by the signal 'in the etheric'! It comes back to the subject of resonance; if the body meets something with which it resonates, a new level of energy can be created. The lithium experiment described on page 14 demonstrates this vital principle.

We can beneficially intervene in hormone secretion and

response to hormones, either by giving potentized hormones or endocrine gland similimums. If the relevant organ can be stimulated, supplementation may indeed be unnecessary. Thyroidea comp. (Heel) is a remedy I have frequent recourse to for treating low energy states, weight problems, putative low thyroid and, surprisingly, it has strong anti-tumour potentiality, since there is a correlation between thyroid disease and cancer. The thyroid has important and generally little-regarded effects in maintaining strong immunity. This is quite logical if you consider that the thyroid is responsible for setting the basal metabolic rate. Often the patient does not need to take thyroxine.

Other possibilities include balancing neuro-transmitters, such as dopamine and serotonin, with consequent benefit to the patient's mental well-being, anti-parasitic programmes and resonance with personal chemical pollution, such as organo-phosphates or heavy metals.

With the benefits of a data file record it is nice to be able to revisit earlier diagnostic discoveries and compare them graphically or numerically with later progress.

TECHNICALITIES

This might be a good moment to consult with the technical boys and ask them the obvious question: how do you get the electronic oscillation 'signature' of, say, serotonin, a vitamin or a pesticide into a computer? It isn't as simple as it sounds. Computers are basically binary bit storage systems, and life is anything but so structured. Certainly Benveniste can do it, since he is digitally recording the resonance harmonics of infra-red radiations (page 130). But this technology has not hitherto been available to the EDS systems manufacturers.

Dr Robert Cass, an EDS specialist from Canada who represents the Avatar EDS system, answered me honestly by saying, 'A little bit of poetry, maybe' (meaning nobody really knows). Dr Julian Kenyon of Southampton, expert with the Vega machine and somewhat opposed to EDS computers, thinks it is nothing more complex than putting the remedy on the test plate and typing in the name on the keyboard.

Vega company are somewhat derisive of other people's technology and claim they have the only legitimate method of
running a disease or remedy signal into an electronic storage system. One may consider this likely to be nothing more than an
assertive marketing stance. One thing is for sure: unless manufacturers come clean, critics will sooner or later find the truth.
It would be a pity to have mud-slinging impair the wider use of
these devices.

CAUSAL CHAINS

I made my reputation as an 'allergy detective'. I've found pathological reactions to all kinds of strange substances, from
herbicide on a bowling ball to a husband's semen, via food,
chemicals, electromagnetic fields and meteorological phenomena. The recoveries have been very gratifying. I hope I will never
lose my knack for this.

But there has always been the nagging question in the background: *why has this person got allergies or intolerances in the
first place?* Part of the ongoing controversy over 25 years of my
clinical ecology practice has been that it is comparatively rare
that these reactions are what I was taught characterized an allergy (IgE-mediated acute hypersensitivity response) when I was at
medical school. It has sometimes been a considerable mystery
why the patient should react as he does. A type of antibody
serum sickness has been proposed, but this is still within the biochemical hypersensitivity domain.

Now at last, since learning EDS, I have begun to find *real* solutions to this riddle. The answers that come up are enlightening,
fascinating, almost unbelievable and, sometimes, rather scary
(see Chapter 12). I have long thought that allergy was really the
final result in the patient's problem, rather than the true cause.
Now I can see that this suspicion is not only well-founded, but I
can get an idea of just how much the patient has suffered, often
without realizing it, to arrive at the doorway marked *'Allergy–
Enter'*.

We speak today of 'causal chains'; that is, the true sequence of
events which led up to the patient's current predicament. The

all-important question, naturally, is *Where did this sequence start?* This often opens the door to a new therapeutic plan which, after all the years of distress and illness, has a good chance of succeeding. It can seem like lateral thinking gone mad sometimes, but there is always an understandable logic behind the events, once they are put into some kind of sequence and perspective.

Nearly always, the problem starts in an unsuspected way with an earlier illness which does not properly resolve. Ed Butler's 'flu of 23 years earlier is just one of many examples. The energetic shadow or disturbance remains in or around the body, sometimes for life, unless it is found and eradicated. One is wise to accept what is found and, time and again, the results speak for the veracity of the hypothesis.

I can only say that I have seen childhood illnesses and especially vaccines initiate disease sequences so many times that I am left with a sense of great unease. What can we do to stop our kids getting ill? I don't think we should abandon the vaccination programmes, we don't want a renewal of the epidemics of old. But how can we get round this difficulty of causing chronic health hazards?

I am not sure. But I do know that my concern is shared by many other doctors who have stumbled across this unpleasant truth while performing routine EAV and EDS. I think that part of the problem is that we *treat* the disease when it manifests and thereby block its proper resolution.

A wise old Chinese doctor, Yang Tschau, once said 'Beware of treating the symptoms of a disease.' Yet in Western biochemically-based medicine that is almost all that is done; no attention is paid to the *true* causes of disease, only the causes of *manifestations* of disease. Yet so often the actual disease is the person's habits and lifestyle; the illness itself is only an outward symptom of what went wrong.

It may emerge in time that it is better to leave most illnesses untreated, especially avoiding the use of allopathic medicines, rather than block natural recovery. I firmly believe from my studies to date that to block an acute illness is to risk driving it underground, from where it may emerge years later to cause a more chronic illness.

Another very worrying concern and challenging management problem is the focus. I already mentioned this phenomenon in Chapter 4; dental foci are discussed further in Chapter 12. It is quite clear to the unprejudiced observer that foci can generate problems far from where they are found. There is compelling evidence that toxic and infective matter can travel along nerve channels, as well as along the more obvious blood route (see page 62). In one case the bacterium *Pseudomonas* was recovered from a cervical spinal osteitis in a man who had the same organism in his urine. The likely mode of travel was along the venous plexus of the spinal column. If this can happen at all, it can happen any time!

I become worried if I think of the bigger implications.

A focus may also pose dangers by initiating pathological changes locally, that is without spreading to a remote site. It is highly likely that an infective focus can give origin to a tumour, possibly due to synthesis of carcinogens by bacterial and fungal micro-organisms. We know that *Aspergillus flavus* (Aflatoxin) and common bacteria, such as *E. coli*, can do this. Late Professor of Neurology in Stockholm Dr Patrick Stortebecker makes it clear that a peri-apical abcess is a very typical finding in close proximity to a jaw cancer.

NEW CLINICAL PERSPECTIVES

It is right to talk about new clinical perspectives with EDS. The whole view of disease changes. Indeed, it is a paradigm shift, no less. Even the language of healing changes. It is proverbial that Eskimos have around 50 words for snow, since their technical knowledge of its form, texture and properties is so much more detailed than ours. It is the same with the new medicine. *Focus, energetic masking, homotoxins* and *mesenchyme* become the new rhetoric, instead of the names of obscure pathogens and weird little eponymous syndromes which most doctors would have to look up in a textbook to remind themselves what form it took.

One becomes confident, I believe, in viewing disease as

non-random but operating to probabilistic laws, governed by energetic phenomena which impact on our physical systems and control them. We are controlled by biological information fields through an energy system; surely this is the way to start looking at disease? Why just mop the floor when you can go back to the leaking tap and turn it off?

Perhaps I can illustrate some of these newer orientations by featuring cases from the files of EDS specialist Ann Smithells, director of the Bio-Tech Health and Nutrition Centre in Petersfield, UK. Ann was a LISTEN user for many years but now has the latest BEST (bio-energetic stress test) system.

Casebook: Male, 53 Years

The patient first attended because of a chemical taste he was experiencing and excreting. His medical history revealed he was taking the medication Sotol for cardiac arrhythmias, he had high stress levels, nausea, headaches, fatigue and lack of concentration.

Ann's initial screening identified Candida, adrenal exhaustion, low zinc and digestive enzymes, plus high levels of toxins in the gall-bladder, prostate, liver, lung and connective tissues. These toxins were mainly heavy metals, probably due to current dental amalgam removal, and very high levels of benzene. The latter was the putative cause of the bad taste.

The patient was given homeopathics and a high dose antioxidant formula to deal with the heavy metal overload and a homeopathic nosode of benzene at 10M and 20X. Four months later he was much improved but there were still high levels of benzene. This forced an investigation into the cause and it turned out to be a leaking fuel pipe in his car, which shunted petrol into the vehicle's ventilation system whenever he pressed the accelerator.

Casebook: Male, 23 Years

The patient attended a year and half after a lengthy tour of the North Vietnam jungle in search of biological specimens. He complained of hunger, significant weight loss, occasional abdominal pain after eating and insufficient energy to participate in sports, despite being a former county tennis player.

Anne identified inflammation of the stomach, liver, lymph meridians (suggesting parasites) and pituitary gland. He also had a high chemical intolerance. A number of exotic parasites were found, together with bacterial encephalitis and high levels of DDT.

The LISTEN system identified the need for 20 different remedies, including nosodes and the miasm Medorrhinum at 10M, and high-dose antioxidants. To complement these therapies the patient was put on a whole-food diet, with lots of organic fruit and vegetables. He was also given a liver support formula, HEP 194 from Biocare, UK.

Within 8 weeks the patient had gained more than a stone (14 lb) in weight and reported his energy was returning to its former levels. Most of the meridians had rebalanced. The liver, which characteristically produces a high reading when detoxing, gradually came down to normal.

This is a patient who had been let down by conventional medicine. It needed a complete rethink from within a different paradigm.

CANCER

It is possible to see cancer coming with good EAV, while it is still just an energy disturbance and sometimes *years* before the actual disease is manifest. Occasionally the EAV cancer-predictive low readings (30 on down) do not show up as expected. It was suggested by EAV expert Anthony Scott-Morley that the tumour may be surrounded by an inflammatory process, which causes paradoxically high readings. However there are a number of warning signs in EDS that would require a high degree of suspicion of cancer, either established or developing imminently. These include readings below 30 on any meridian, multiple large ID drops, high biological age, low immune performance, chronic toxic overload, dangerous foci in the teeth and anaerobic burdenings (meaning that the general cell chemistry is running too slowly and not burning up molecular fuel properly, creating toxins).

Probably there is no better way of summarizing the difference between the methods of the EDS prescriber and the conventional doctor than to review cancer therapy. Western scientific doctors look upon cancer as an invasion; cancer cells are 'the enemy'. Their response is to fight back with as much fire power as possible, in an attempt to slaughter every last cancer cell. The patient's body becomes the battlefield and is otherwise ignored. Yet anyone who has seen pictures of the blasted wastelands around the trenches of the First World War will know that the battlefield comes off worse than either army.

The EDS specialist looks at cancer as the final results of many disease pathways. We are used to thinking of it as a tissue ageing process, where toxins and pathogens have accumulated to such an extent that the body defences can no longer cope. We try to undo the ill-effects of years of negative health, thread by thread.

Douglas Lieber, director of Computronix Electromedical Systems and the inventor of the Acupro system, pinpoints seven main factors contributing to deterioration in health and leading, if untreated, ultimately to system breakdown and the threat of cancer. These are:

1 geopathic stress, centred especially around the patient's bed or daytime chair
2 parasites of many types present in the body
3 degenerative toxic focus, most commonly in the teeth or jaws but also often in the tonsils or pelvic abdominal areas
4 unresolved emotional trauma
5 miasmic influences, from parent to child, passed through the generations
6 radiation and/or electromagnetic exposure
7 personal chemical pollution with toxins such as nickel,

cadmium, mercury, aflatoxins (from moulds and fungi), pesticides, benzene, toluene, xylene, formaldehyde, isopropyl alcohol and 'autotoxins', chiefly from the patient's own intestines.[2]

EDS specialists make no attempts to treat the cancer, only to treat the patient. If he or she is going to survive the intruder, the patient will need a fortified immune system that is capable of closing down the attack. This can only be achieved by detoxing, removing coincidental and distracting pathology, pumping up nutrition and taking remedies known to stimulate immunity. Of course this cannot all be done with homeopathy. I myself give intravenous drips containing high-key nutritional supplements, especially high-dose vitamin C which is a proven safe cytotoxic agent. Dental work and other physical intervention may be indicated.

Most important of all, *the patient must change his or her life, radically.* Cancer is a wake-up call; it means the patient is badly off-balance in respect of all or part of his or her life. Unless steps are taken to remedy toxic relationships, unhappy work conditions and low self-image, then no therapy is going to be effective against cancer.

It is hardly necessary to point out that these are good universal health measures and apply to any chronic disease process. I call it my ortho-immune programme.

CHAPTER 9

LIGHT AS THERAPY

It is important not to forget that light is just another electromagnetic wave form. The fact that we can see it gives us a deep psychological relationship to light; but it is really no different in quality to radio-waves or x-rays. Because of this we can gain a glimpse of what detailed information may be contained in energy form.

Among the earliest writers to advocate the medical use of light were Herodotus, Galen and the great Arabian physician Avicenna. The ancient Egyptians used a type of colour therapy. But the Greeks went further in both the theory and practice of light medicine, using the sun's rays to treat disease in the famous healing temples of Heliopolis (Sun City).

In our own century, Nobel Laureate Albert Szent-Gyorgi, who discovered vitamin C, acknowledges the profound influence of light on our health and states 'all the energy we take into our bodies is derived from the sun.'[1] By this he means that light is turned from electromagnetic sun energy into energized chemicals by the process of photosynthesis in plants. These plant energy substances (food) are subsequently taken in by leaf-eating animals, who are then in turn devoured by carnivorous species. Ultimately, all life energy derives from the sun. It is correct to speak of light as a *nutrient*.

But Szent-Gyorgi took it much further than this. His research concluded that many of the body's enzymes and hormones are functionally sensitive to light. Colour changes can significantly affect the power and effectiveness of these enzymes and hormones. His findings were subsequently verified by researchers Martinek and Berezin in 1979. They found that some colours can increase the activity of enzymes by up to 500 per cent and markedly affect the transport of chemicals across cell membranes.[2] It has even been found that the absence of certain wavelengths in light results in the body being unable to absorb fully all dietary nutrients.

Little wonder, then, that *lack* of light can have severely destructive health consequences. Few people today have not heard of the unfortunate condition of SAD, or Seasonal Affect Disorder. This is a disorder in which the shortage of adequate sunlight during the winter months of a northern climate causes gradual loss of vitality and even suicidal depression. The cure, quite naturally, is to enhance ambient light levels, either by judiciously taken winter holidays in sunnier climes, or the artificial simulation of daylight. This can be supplied by means of lamps with an adjusted output that has the correct natural daylight spectrum of colours (normal electric lighting has far too much of the yellow frequencies and is lacking in red and blue-violet).

BIOPHOTONS

In 1923 the Russian scientist Alexander Gurwitsch speculated that cells contained light energy. He placed the roots of two onion shoots very close together and noted that they had a positive effect on each other's growth. If he separated them by means of a glass partition, this mutual synergy did not take place; however, if the dividing screen was made of quartz, the original mutual benefit was once again manifest. Gurwitsch concluded therefore that the growth influence had something to do with ultra-violet light emitted by the roots.

In 1982 biophysicist Fritz Popp finally proved the existence of light emitted by living plant cells, in a series of experiments using a residual light amplifier at the Max Planck Institute of Astronomy in Heidelberg. Popp went further and recognized that the intensity of the signal was not critical, but the *frequency* and what is termed *coherence* were.[3] Coherent light has a high degree of order and this is the equivalent of making it more 'intense' since the wave peaks occur together and reinforce each other.

What Popp showed was that clearer and more vigorous light emissions are associated with rapid growth, whereas this falls away with cell ageing. He also found that when cells die they give off a flash of light which must have somehow been stored within the cell. He coined the term 'biophotons' for light of this order. DNA seems to be the origin of these photons. Perhaps most remarkable of all was the discovery that when an organism dies almost all its cells give up their 'death flash' at the same moment, some eight hours after the cessation of apparent life.

The New Age idea that we are light beings somehow now doesn't seem quite so improbable! Clearly life values and light are inseparable. This argues that light has considerable power for healing, reinforcing the subjective beliefs of many energy healing practitioners. It also follows that lack of light, especially the coherent sort, is a contributory factor in diseases.

MAL-ILLUMINATION

The study of light adaptation in humans and the attendant ills caused by deficiencies or incorrect balance in colour frequencies has gone on apace in the last few decades. We now have the term *mal-illumination*, a concept proposed by John Nash Ott, who works with therapeutic full-spectrum lighting.[4] He compares this term with our existing term 'malnutrition'. Windows, windscreens, eyeglasses and urban pollution are among the factors which alter the nature of the light our bodies receive, by filtering out some of the wavelengths. Mal-illumination is said to contribute to fatigue, tooth decay, depression, hostility, suppressed immune function, strokes, loss of hair, skin damage and even cancer.

Sunlight is therefore vital to our well-being and, in the current climate of ultraviolet scares, this should not be lost sight of (no pun intended). Despite the medical fad for claiming that skin cancer is caused by sunlight, the evidence points in exactly the opposite direction. A paper published in the 7th August 1982 edition of the British medical journal the *Lancet*, based on a study carried out jointly between the London School of Hygiene and Tropical Medicine and the University of Sydney's Melanoma Clinic, found that the incidence of malignant melanoma was far higher in office workers than in those who were regularly exposed to sunlight due to lifestyle or occupation.[5]

When scientific opinion departs from common sense, it is nearly always science that is found wrong in the end. In this case it is *dangerously* wrong! Light simply cannot be both a nutrient and a poison at normal ambient levels.

CEREBRAL PATHWAYS

The fact is that most of today's light therapy work, colour therapies included, is concerned with light delivered to the eyes. It travels the optic pathways and stimulates, among other regions, the hypothalamus, which is part of the endocrine system and thus influences a most all bodily functions. It seems likely, in the light of modern research, that the pineal gland is far from the vestigial organ it was once thought to be but is actually a master gland which regulates the body's circadian rhythms. As befits the 'Third Eye', it is truly light-sensitive and once again the quality of light received is the crucial factor in maintaining the delicate impulses that regulate the fundamental balance of functions and maintain health.

LIGHT TO THE TISSUES

Light is of unquestionable value via the optical nerve route, as the growing body of scientific evidence and clinical experience shows. But revolutionary healing work with light energy radiation delivered directly to the stressed tissues using machines which deliver quantum 'excited' gem substances, such as diamond and sapphire, is one of the most fascinating and promising frontiers of medicine.

Probably the most advanced machine of this type is the Lux Caduceus III, developed by Jon Whale of Arnside in Cumbria. An electronic design engineer by profession, in the 1980s he designed electronic transducers using emeralds and blue sapphires and used them to cure a number of cases of psoriasis and chronic cystitis. He now runs a busy practice in the north of England and manufactures his equipment for world-wide export. He now runs a busy practice in the north of England and manufactures his equipment for world-wide export.

The essence of this approach is that light can be 'stressed' with the characteristics of the gems. The changes to the light are probably at the quantum level and we are unable to perceive them. But the body tissues can detect the changes and react differently to each type of light, in a most remarkable and consistent fashion.

The important point to grasp is that light travels very far into the tissues. The experience of shining a torch through your hand on a dark night will tell you this; even a small wattage of a 3 volt battery torch will make the back of the hand glow red as the blood vessels and deep tissue are illuminated. The Caduceus Lux lamps use high-intensity bulbs. The powerful beam is filtered and focused through lenses and consequently has far more penetration. Whale has designed lamps which house the gems in the path of the light and concentrate it in a useful beam. The whole apparatus is simple to use and, indeed, a number of users are paramedical in status only, yet obtain results that are little short of sensational. Recoveries range from breast lumps to arthritis, eczema to colitis.

AYURVEDIC GEM ELIXIR THERAPY

This whole new science is really an extension of existing ayurvedic gem elixir therapy, which has a long and distinguished tradition in the Indian subcontinent and can be traced back to Egyptian times. Gems are placed into the tincture liquid and the whole exposed to sunlight until the elixir takes on the characteristics of that gem substance. Theory views disease and disharmony as basically colour starvation; the 'excited' liquid of the elixir rectifies the energy deficit.[6]

As Whale explains, the huge bejewelled rings that were worn by Indian princes, nabobs and potentates were not always merely for the display of wealth and self-aggrandisement. Some rings were intended for therapeutic purposes. Such a ring had no back, so that sunlight could shine straight through the precious stone and so irradiate the skin and tissues beneath with beneficial rays (in common with all energy medicine systems, it is not necessary to bathe the whole body in the treatment or remedy in order to benefit from it).

The other major traditional route of administration was using ground-up gem powders. I consider this a very dangerous practice and it is not to be recommended. It is wrong and over-simplifies the case to feel that gems are safe just because they are manifestly not *chemically* toxic or come from an esoteric background. These substances can be very powerful emanators and modulators of quantum electromagnetic force, as we shall see below, and should be regarded seriously as such. Introducing solid substances which perhaps may never be removed or excreted fully from the body, but can go on causing harm if they are the wrong choice, may prove disastrous. Even when we understand these things much better than we do now, it still lacks sensible rationale as these gem powders may pre-empt any possibility of changing modalities as the body's state or disease process alters.

Readers who wish to experiment with gem elixirs should make them up as described above and *not* take the solid form – even if cost is no object!

Gem Science

Unfortunately, this fascinating yet cogent discipline has too long languished and is still little known outside its country of origin. Modern light therapists and researchers such as Jacob Liberman and John Ott seem to ignore it. But with the advancement of science and the ability to translate older methods from a stultifying background into a modern framework and quantifiable results, we may say 'gem therapy' has indeed come of age and will grow steadily in applications in the West.

Despite superficial similarities, this is not crystal therapy. Quartz, amethyst, tourmaline, moonstone and many other commonly used therapeutic crystals the reader may have heard about seem to have little or no value in this 'light-stressing' context.

Nor is it exactly colour therapy. Tests show that the colour of the light is irrelevant. In other words, it is the *gem* which dictates the resulting effect and not its colour as perceived by the patient. This is odd, since the Indian tradition regards the need for gems and their effectiveness as being evidence of colour starvation.

Notwithstanding, Whale adds the colours traditionally associated with each gem (see list below). But he emphasizes that these colour filters could be dispensed with. The gem carries the energy signal. Whale also electronically modulates the gem stones in his lamps with an additional frequency associated with the body's own natural healing frequencies.

What you feel when you put your hand in the beam is a distinct and palpable pressure from the radiation. It is an astonishing thing to experience. Light from the Caduceus III has the power to shine right through the skull or chest and will thus reach all tissues, even bone, though in varying intensity according to its density.

The applications are remarkably diverse. Thus emerald and sapphire, when excited, emit cooling soothing energies which can stop eczema or inflammation dead in their tracks. Focused on the bowel, this represents a totally new method of calming the gut in, say, colitis or diverticulitis. Ruby will energize cells and glands, and Whale asserts it is excellent for rejuvenating tired male potency. Diamond, on the other hand, is stimulating and, mixed with yellow citrine, peps up lethargy and fatigue states such as those which characterize ME, Candida and complex allergy conditions. But too much diamond can cause a patient to lose sleep for several days.

The principal effect of the main gems and their associated colours are shown here:

Gem	Colour	Energy Output and Properties
Carnelian	Orange	*Cooling, moist and harmonizing, anti-allergic*
Chrysoberyl	Infrared	*Hot, penetrating, cleansing, deep heating*
Citrine	Yellow	*Warm, enlivening, cleansing*
Diamond	Indigo	*Stimulating, invigorating, clarifying, antidepressant*
Emerald	Green	*Cold, unifying and solidifying, analgesic*
Ruby	Red	*Heating, drying, energizing, expanding*

Sapphire	Violet	*Tranquillizing, soothing, analgesic, antispasmodic*
Topaz	Blue	*Cool, soft, satisfying, antiseptic*

Combinations

Traditional ayurvedic gem therapy includes the use of certain combinations of gems. Sure enough, these too are effective when supplied electronically. Thus emerald and sapphire make an excellent combination which is cooling, soothing and analgesic. Carnelian and diamond through the chest is a good combination for asthma, to allergically cleanse and energize the struggling lungs. Obesity might be benefited by ruby and diamond, to increase heat and stimulate blood flow, especially if directed to the thyroid to increase metabolism.

Two classical compound mixtures frequently used are IBGO (Indigo-Blue-Green-Orange) or, in other words, diamond-topaz-emerald-carnelian, and the so-called 'Seven Gems' mix which combines all the principal stones except chrysoberyl. These can be used when the picture is complicated, uncertain or simply in cases where generalized light and energy support therapy is needed.

Some conditions, and their suggested gem treatments, are given here and should make the overall principles clear:

Acne	Citrine/Topaz
Alopecia	Sapphire
Anaemia	Ruby
Arthritis	Sapphire/Emerald
Asthma	Carnelian/Diamond
Bronchitis	Citrine/Diamond
Burns	Emerald
Cystitis	Emerald
Conjunctivitis	Carnelian
Constipation	Citrine
Depression	Diamond
Debility	Ruby/Diamond
Diabetes	Diamond/Citrine
Diarrhoea	Emerald

Eczema	Emerald/Sapphire
Epilepsy	Diamond
Gastritis	Emerald
Headache	Sapphire
Insomnia	Sapphire
Irritable bowel	Emerald/Sapphire
Menopause	Carnelian
Migraine	Sapphire
Pain	Sapphire/Emerald
Pleurisy	Topaz
Psoriasis	Sapphire
Rheumatism	Ruby/Sapphire
Sciatica	Sapphire
Shingles	Sapphire/Emerald
Sterility	Diamond
Stomach ulcer	Emerald/Sapphire
Tonsillitis	Topaz
Varicose ulcer	Ruby/Diamond

ELECTRONIC FREQUENCY

There is another dimension completely in this unique Virtual Energy therapy. Because of the introduction of Western electronic technology we are able to add a pulsed frequency to the healing rays. This can enormously influence the power and range of effects. For example, a frequency of 3.3 Hertz (Hz) is identical to the brainwave pattern known as theta, which is associated with trance and dreamlike states (see list of brainwave frequencies, below). If we take emerald and sapphire light and beam it into the skull at 3.3 Hz, the results are quite dramatic. The subject will rapidly descend into a beautiful dreamlike trance, which is very potent at countering stress. We call this *samadhi*, an Indian word meaning 'bliss', which gives a fair description of its subjective result. I use it before all other treatments on my own Caduceus. I argue that all patients are stressed and miserable by virtue of being ill, and this wonderful eased state of mind is a very sound concomitant treatment. The effect lasts up to 24 hours, sometimes longer.

Other useful frequencies are 8 Hz, the Earth's own 'Gaia' resonant frequency, and around 1.5 – 2.5 Hz, which is the lowest band, delta brainwaves. The latter frequency accords with deep unconsciousness and therefore has analgesic potential, rather like an anaesthetic. Combined with soothing emerald it can work wonders for bruised tissue or painful joints.

Logically, diamond would be coupled with 15 – 20 Hz, which is low beta. We never use high beta (above 25 Hz), which is excessively stimulating, since all healing requires calm and ease.

Rhythm	Frequency	State of Consciousness
High beta	above 25 Hz	*Anxiety, panic, anger, psychosis*
Beta	14 – 25 Hz	*Attention focuses on external affairs, 'normal waking'*
Alpha	7.8 – 14 Hz	*Relaxed, attention divided between internal and external matters*
Theta	3.2 – 7.8 Hz	*Dreaming, trance, hypnosis, internal attention*
Delta	01. – 3.2	*Deep sleep, unconsciousness, coma*

As with all advanced technology, the degree of success with the equipment depends considerably on the knowledge and competence of the practitioner. Whereas anyone can get basic results of value, if the use of electronic gem therapy is combined with a good working knowledge of the alternative models, many possibilities open up. For example, eczema is often a symptom of gut overload, especially liver toxicity ('liver anger'). Therefore supporting energies at, say, Gaia frequency to the liver can be an excellent complement to the direct use of soothing emerald light onto the skin.

Carnelian and diamond is an ideal mixture for the circulation and lymph system (8 Hz) and can be used in many ways, for example in the treatment of varicose ulcer or dependant oedema

– the latter can be viewed by the layman as an inefficient heart pumping action. But this mixture can create healing pathways at many deeper levels. Thus diamond and carnelian to the spleen area can produce a dramatic benefit for the immune system, resulting in improvement or elimination of many complex allergies. Whale even reports the resolution of two lymphoma cases (malignant condition of lymphoid tissue).

I myself use the mixtures known as VIBGYOR or 'Seven Gems' to the thymus, since this gland is associated with white cell education and maturity and I am deeply involved with the immune system, being known primarily as an allergist. In addition to detox and homeopathic cleansing of the intercellular tissues, this is of great benefit to the chronically ill patient.

Whale's Caduceus equipment has the further refinement of multiple channels. More than one lamp can be rigged and used simultaneously. Thus, for example, the deeply relaxing *samadhi* can be administered at the same time as other specific organ therapy. Or a stimulating mixture at energizing frequencies can be shone into the thymus gland at the same time that soothing emerald and carnelian at theta are used on allergic eczema of the lower leg.

Electronic gem therapy also lends itself very well to being combined with other healing models. Instead of organ or tissue support therapy, excited light can be used to enhance or 'open' chakras. This is the basis of Whale's claim for enhancing male potency. He has discovered that a series of treatments using ruby light to the base chakra has a powerful stimulating effect and is certainly safer and preferable to modern drug and psychotherapy prescriptions for this commoner-than-supposed condition. Diamond and topaz to the throat chakra will sometimes produce an immediate change in voice and expression, and 'Seven Gems' to the heart chakra is the nearest thing we have to a treatment for lost love and the pain of separation.

Naturally, this is further support for the validity and existence of chakras since they can be positively influenced in this way, the results becoming unarguably manifest in *this* reality.

Potentized Water

There is a return to the tradition of gem elixirs, using the Caduceus lamps to excite alcohol and water with the properties of the gems. This is essentially the same idea as the old method of preparing therapeutic elixirs, which was to put the gem in a mother tincture and expose the whole to several weeks of sunlight. We ought perhaps to keep in mind that Indian sunlight is a good deal more brilliant than ours in northern Europe. Whale's lamps may be the only truly effective way of preparing such medicines at these latitudes.

On a purely anecdotal level, I can vouch for the effectiveness of these simple medicines. A glass of 'diamond water', which after all costs much the same as tap water, can dispel sleep for many hours and sometimes even result in serious insomnia. It can be a writer's boon and far less damaging than the many caffeine stimulant drinks to which many youngsters are now addicted.

Casebook: Female, 45 Years

A woman therapist had torn a muscle in an amateur stage production. The noise of the muscle rupture was so loud it was heard in the second row. She was promptly incapacitated and in great pain.

She came to see me a few days later, limping badly, all other attempts at therapy having failed. I gave her first a routine 20 minutes of *samadhi*, with emerald-sapphire stones at 3.3 Hz. This very aware patient was able to tell me that her pelvis underwent a shift back into the normal energetic position during this stage.

I followed through with about 30 minutes to the injured calf. All pain had now vanished from the affected leg, but now a new pain had appeared in the opposite knee. This was probably due to the stress of limping and bearing all her weight on that side, but the pain had, of necessity, been suppressed. The lamps had probably melted away the suppressing energy shield.

A further 15 minutes on the uninjured side removed that discomfort too, and the patient walked to her car with no discernible limp. Next day she phoned to say there was only mild discomfort, she was back at work and she was content with just one treatment.

Casebook: Male, 6 Years

This boy had been diagnosed as having disintegrative psychosis, a variety of autism which I have long suspected comes on after vaccination, particularly for measles. My reasoning was as follows: an autistic youngster seems to be very 'out of contact' and 'dreamy'; he (they are usually males) is very introverted into the right brain hemisphere. If we can use the gem therapy to accelerate the left brain and inhibit right-brain activity, we may be able to wake up his logical and reasoning faculties.

Accordingly, I put him on a one-week programme of diamond, citrine and ruby to the left cranial hemisphere and emerald-sapphire to the right brain. I further refined this strategy by using beta (high brain activity) of around 15 Hz to the left side and a retarding and soothing 3.3 Hz to the right hemisphere. I lowered the penetration to minimal wattage in order not to 'cross-over' and inadvertently stimulate the opposite side, or vice versa.

Within days he began vocalizing well and within a month was forming intelligible sentences. For a number of reasons he was unable to continue any further treatments with the Caduceus Lux III, but despite this he continued to make rapid progress. He has learned to use a computer keyboard and happily spends hours amusing himself with electronic games, which of course require considerable left-brain dexterity. His mother reports he has learned to integrate well with his peers. One year later I had a report he is now regraded as mentally normal for schooling purposes.

One of my major plans for the future is to explore this healing route for autism.

BIOLUMANETICS

Nature has the endless capacity to surprise and fascinate us. Biolumanetics, a new science of healing, is just about the most unusual medical application of light in therapy I have heard of. The system was developed by a 62-year-old American engineer called Patrick Richards. In 1983 he designed an instrument called a Luminator™ which balances air temperatures for efficient office energy management. In fact his invention turned out to have a far more important and totally novel application than the one for which it was made.

While testing the unit in an open plan office, Richards found that many people reported unexpected health gains, from reduction of stress and migraine levels to disappearance of low back pain. The big question was – *Why?*

The Luminator™ alters the local environment in three main ways:

1 Temperatures are balanced uniformly throughout (wall-to-wall, floor-to-ceiling).
2 An altered magnetic field is created.
3 The available light in the room is altered from incoherent (light going in many directions) to coherent (polarized into one plane only).

In 1985 Richards discovered by serendipity that light from living cell forms could be imaged in the field of the Luminator™. Late 1985 found him photographing people holding their medications and noting how, as Abrams and Voll had discovered before, that the patient's energy status alters for the better dramatically. In the case of Richards' equipment, a sick person may have a very blurred, indistinct image, but simply by holding an effective medication the person's special photographic image becomes immediately sharp and clear. Logically, if the medication is not suitable, the image remains blurred or becomes even more foggy.

Subsequently, Richards went on to develop a unique and sophisticated method of assessing patients and establishing suitable remedies. He calls his system VRIC (visual reference of image coherence) and it basically entails the use of enhanced photography to measure the vitality and coherence of any life form — human, plant or animal. To make a VRIC assessment image requires a fixed focus Polaroid camera and the Luminator™ as a source. The brightness, intensity and coherence of the light reflected by the patient and captured on the photograph is a precise indication of his or her health and energy status. Therapy would then consist of taking a base image and endeavouring to find a remedy, or more than one remedy, which will make it sharper and brighter, much as the EAV practitioner does by eliminating the ID drop.

Arguably this is a milestone development for practitioners in the field of energetic healing, indeed all therapeutic practice. We can now see objective changes after Reiki, homeopathy, flower essences, shiatsu and colour therapy, to name just a few.

Again, the vital side of the body energy information field is made abundantly clear: the medication need only be put on the floor close to the subject to transmit its signal. No contact is required, but provided it is within the energetic aura the light coherence may change markedly. No smoke, no mirrors! That's about as much 'proof' as we have for you at present of the tenets of energy healing expounded in these pages.

A patient can of course bring his or her own medication for assessment, but VRIC specialists have their own repertoire of preferences and a range of special frequencies called 'Lumanetics' which Richards claims are not affected by Gaia fields. When a suitable therapeutic match is made, the 'vibrational signature' is transferred to an anionic chelate fluid, which is a negatively-charged fluid made in a special field. It is said not only to hold the required therapeutic energy but actually to bind magnetically with toxins and impurities in order to help them be eliminated,[7] though I find statements like this hard to take without some experimental support.

Probably the most exciting potential of all with the VRIC system is in assessing the energy dynamics of interpersonal relationships. The photograph can tell a person if the partner he or she is with is 'right' for them or not. The common complaint 'I feel really drained with that person' can now be expressed in an objective and impersonal way. With a stressful individual standing in close proximity to the subject, the assessment image is blurred, whereas with other neutral companions it remains relatively sharp. It is remarkable to reflect just how radical a change it could bring to our turbulent over-emotional society to be able to assess family, love relationships, professional and personal relationships (in fact any relationship at all) in a clear, precise and *non-judgemental* manner.

On a recent visit to the practice facility of Thrity Engineer, a London-based practitioner of Biolumanetics, I was shown several fascinating examples of family group dynamics. In one instance, a child taking Ritalin for ADD (attention deficit disorder) was quite coherent without the medicine. When his sibling and father stood next to him, he remained fully coherent. But as soon as his mother joined the group, the child's image went incoherent. The surprising course of action was therefore to given the *mother* a remedy, which made the boy coherent again when she held it. The mother was subsequently treated and the boy recovered completely, without any further need of medication.

Thrity also showed me what Richards calls right-and-left-brain-coherence. This is accessed by photographing the patient with the left eye open, right eye closed and then vice versa. An individual will sometimes be incoherent in one modality but not the other.

Casebook: Female, 43 Years

A woman was distressed by the loss of her son some years before. When she held a photograph of the deceased in her right hand (left brain), she remained coherent. But when the photograph was put in her left hand (right brain) she became quite visually incoherent. It is easy to see that she could rationalize her loss (left brain logic) but could not come to terms with the emotions (right brain).

A suitable remedy was chosen photographically and her emotional patterns changed at once to a better and healthier regard for her lost offspring.

Incidentally, I was fascinated to see that even the house-plants which appear in Thrity's photographs would become incoherent along with an incoherent human source nearby. But recovered fully next to a healthy individual!

Biolumanetics claims not to address directly the symptoms of illness. There is nothing to tell the practitioner at what level the bio-energetic disturbance lies, whether energetic, emotional or physical. Thus the approach question is not 'What is causing this incoherence?' but 'What will make this system vital or coherent?'

As Thrity Engineer says, 'Accuracy, specificity, precision and safety are the hallmarks of the VRIC assessment system. The photos can't lie.'[8] No doubt we will all hear more of the Biolumanetics system in the future.

CHAPTER 10

GAIA

This is a book about human health and the biological significance of electromagnetism and other energy forces in diagnosis and healing. Quantum potential fields are invoked to explain some of the stranger manifestations which can be observed objectively. But in this chapter we must make the point that we are all subject to much larger energy influences, which are great in magnitude and inescapable by life on Earth. I am referring to the Earth's own energies.

Those of us who care about such things think a lot about the extent to which our lives are influenced by the field phenomena from the 'Earth Mother' or Gaia, as Richard Lovelock called it. A few years ago it would have been regarded as absurd to consider that the Earth's magnetic field could possibly have an effect on a mammalian species such as humans. Today the only intelligent question, and an important one, is: How could the Earth's electromagnetic energy field possibly *not* have a profound influence on our biology and health?

It is absurd to suppose that this rich and enormous variable energy field has no relevance to our well-being. We may feel we are important from our own limited perspective, but on the bigger scale of things we are quite inconsequential, in orders of magnitude, compared to the Earth's overwhelmingly greater presence. Just because we have hitherto had no awareness of the phenomenon and no satisfactory means of measuring its biological effects does not mean these don't exist. We have been naïve for far too long. It has become increasingly clear that Gaia is a health issue, as well as an ecological one. Remember Abrams' reflex (where neurologist Albert Abrams noticed a strange dull percussion note when tapping certain areas of his patients' abdomens, which turned up not only in cancer and tuberculosis cases, but even in healthy patients situated in close proximity to cancer or tuberculosis specimens – see Chapter 1). The *big* clue here was the fact that the critical diagnosis could only be made with the patient oriented east—west.

There is a newly-emerged phenomenon we call geopathic stress, meaning that there are certain spots on the Earth which are unhealthy due to distortion of the Earth's field at that point. Many patients will not respond to treatment, particularly any that relies on manipulation of biological energy such as most of the natural therapies, unless any pre-existing geopathic stress is removed.

But the issue is far bigger than this, as we shall see.

THE EARTH'S FIELD

The earth's core is a spinning mass of molten iron. It sets up a huge magnetic field (known variably as the geomagnetic field or magnetosphere), which merges at the poles and spreads out into space for thousands of kilometres. But this field in turn is greatly influenced by an even more powerful energy field: that of the sun. We speak today of 'solar wind', which means the outpourings of charged electrical particles streaming into space with incredible energies, pushing matter before it (there is enough force to propel a rocket up to nearly the speed of light, given time). Most of the force is dissipated into empty regions, but where it meets the magnetic field of a planet, such as the Earth, there are considerable interactions.

On the solar side of the Earth the geomagnetic field is compressed by the pressure of particles and radiation travelling at or near the speed of light. On the far side, the geomagnetic field is thrust far out into space. Certain regions on the sunward side are 'sandwich layers' where high-energy particles are trapped, bouncing around endlessly and forming a kind of cushion. These layers are called the Van Allen belts, after their discoverer. If it were not for the presence of the Van Allen belts, absorbing and damping radiation, life on Earth would be totally unsustainable, except far underground.

Solar wind

Compressed
magnetic field

Van Allen belts

Magnetotail

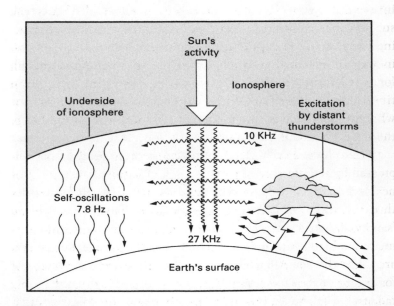

Sun's
activity

Ionosphere

Underside
of ionosphere

Excitation
by distant
thunderstorms

10 KHz

Self-oscillations
7.8 Hz

27 KHz

Earth's surface

It comes as a shock to realize that our friendly sun's rays are so deadly to life. Astronauts can only survive for short periods in space without being shielded, and rocket missions are carefully timed to avoid maximum solar radiation. Outside the Earth's protective magnetosphere humans would be sizzled if they chanced to be caught in a solar storm. I make this point in the hope that it gives a vivid picture of the hostility of the sun's radiation and what we would potentially face down here on the surface, if our protection should fail.

The sun has great power for health and healing, but it would be absurd to think it was not capable of an adverse influence, even at the radiation levels we experience.

ELECTRICAL FIELD

The Earth's magnetosphere does not rotate because the sun's forces grip it. Instead the planetary rook-and-iron ball rotates once every 24 hours within the vast energy shell. On the principle of a dynamo, this generates enormous electrical charges, in the range of billions of watts, even when the sun is quiescent. It is as if we were living inside a cosmically-scaled electrical machine. The dynamo effect also results in ionizing radiation (the deadly radiation of atomic bombs) and extremely low-frequency (ELF) radiation which causes strange and unhealthy biological disturbances.

Any particular spot on the Earth's surface passes through the magnetic field once every 24 hours, from high to low and back again, giving us our basic diurnal variations. It is more important than light levels, and because of it the passage of day can be felt even in total darkness.

Considering the dangerous highly charged natural environment in which we live, it stands to reason that life has evolved very precariously. We could all be snuffed out like the dinosaurs at any moment. But this also tells us that life here is, for the present, cleverly adapted to this background radiation. Provided the variations are not too large, we can accommodate them.

However, there are times when the sun erupts into extra activity. At these times, the powers unleashed are almost unimaginable to us. The intensity of the solar wind rises and the dangers from the emissions are obviously increased many-fold. The beautiful aurorae or flickering coloured sheets of light in the polar night skies are one of the relatively fortunate consequences. More problematical is the widespread disruption of computers, navigational equipment and telecommunications apparatus.

Fortunately this is not too common an occurrence. But it is hardly surprising, in view of the brain's electrical properties, that at these times people's behaviour may become disturbed. It isn't common knowledge, but there is a marked rise in psychiatric hospital admissions at times of peak sunspot activity. This statistic alone makes it clear that the sun's rays can be bad for us and that Gaia isn't all sweetness and light.

MAGNETIC REVERSALS

The truth is, we have survived on Earth partly because of and partly despite the sun's influence. There are worrying events in the past which may dent the 'friendly goddess' Gaia image. Every once in a while the Earth's magnetic field undergoes a tremendous upheaval and reverses itself; north pole to south and vice versa. Typically these transformations have taken around 10,000 years, which might seem a long time to a human but is a mere blink of an eye in geological terms. Nobody knows why these cataclysmic reversals take place, but one thing is very clear: they are deadly to life, leading to widespread extinction of species, particularly animal life. This is probably because the magnetosphere dies away during the transition and the protective fields such as the Van Allen belts cease to shield the planetary surface from the ferocity of the sun's radiation.

As an aside, these mass die-offs make nonsense out of Darwinian evolution, though some scientists have tried to explain the discrepancies of Darwin's theories by inventing 'punctuated equilibrium'. By this contrivance the theory of a slow, tortured evolution is kept alive. Once Vitalism (see Chapter 1) is understood and embraced, these crutches to mechanistically-conceived life will prove unnecessary.

Is this phenomenon of reversal relevant to us? Well, we cannot predict – as we can with the mathematical probability that the next major meteorite impact is actually long overdue – when the next magnetic field reversal will take place. Contemporary measurements tell us that the intensity of the Earth's field has been on the wane for several decades. But Robert Becker writes that this is largely an academic matter: we have produced far more than the equivalent of a magnetic field reversal by virtue of the magnetic outpourings that Man himself has created.[1] Becker calls it electro-pollution. We have created our own dangerous environment and it is already having a health impact.

ARTIFICIAL RADIATION

Most people overlook the fact that microwaves and radio waves are part of the electromagnetic spectrum, parts of which are deadly (x-rays, alpha rays and gamma rays). The medical profession was caught off-guard too, and for a time microwave heating of the tissues (diathermy) was considered an excellent treatment for a wide variety of conditions. Just what microwaves are capable of is seen clearly by the effect on a good steak.

But just because radio waves carry our favourite television programmes and news of The Lottery does not mean they are safe. In fact we are now exposed to a combined radiation exposure from all sources which exceeds a million-fold the natural background radiation in which we evolved as a species. It has now become a dominant health issue, implicated in causing some childhood leukaemias, suicides, heart disease, maybe sudden infant death syndrome, and probably many other conditions that have not been reported because the connection has not been made yet (my views on cot death are different and clearly expressed in my last book *The Complete Guide to Food Allergy and Environmental Illness*).[2]

This remains a contentious issue, but one thing is clear; experiments show that our immune systems are adversely influenced at radiation levels far lower than we are currently exposed to. As I described in my last book, experiments on animals have shown that T-cell function can be harmed by very low levels of microwaves and therefore lose their ability to recognize cancer cells and other invaders. Tests at the College of Pharmacy in Illinois have shown that lymphoid organs subjected to magnetic resonance go into a leukaemia-like state (a drop in white blood cells but no effect on red blood cells) which is reversible when the current ceases. Work at the School of Aerospace Medicine in Houston, Texas, showed that radio frequencies alter the immune system. Could this have anything to do with the fact that amateur radio enthusiasts have triple the normal incidence of myeloid leukaemia? Common sense says it could. The inevitable result of impaired immune function is chronic fatigue syndrome and the increased risk of cancer. The disturbing thing about these tests is that exposures were well within the range that might be found in any typical modern home (see below).

The worst type of radiation to be exposed to is that we call extremely low frequency fields (ELFs); these are in the range 10–150 Hertz. These cause the most harm biologically. It is ironic that the domestic electricity supply in most Western countries is set at 50–60 Hz, ensuring that most appliances give off a dangerous magnetic flux. Robert Becker points out that cancer cells exposed to a frequency of 60 Hz undergo a transformation and multiply at over 1,600 times the normal rate, making them far more deadly than 'normal' cancer cells.

Typical levels of ambient alternating electrical fields in our environment are shown here:[3]

Location	Range (volts/m^2)
Home/office background	0.9–10
VDU at 50 cm	2–90
Close to domestic appliance	6–200
Industrial background	10–400
Under large power line	500–3,000
Power station near generator	1,000–5,000
Electrical field during a thunderstorm	1,000–50,000

Remember also that some unpleasant effects from electricity supply may be due to low-frequency sound vibrations, caused by resonance with the mains frequency. The buzzing of fluorescent tubes is a case in point. Sound waves have a distinct pressure that is capable of great harm to biological systems.

Safe Dosage Levels

According to Becker, all abnormal man-made electromagnetic fields, regardless of their frequencies, are potentially harmful biologically. He lists the resultant effects as follows:

1 effects on growing cells, such as increases in the rate of cancer-cell division
2 increases in the incidence of certain cancers
3 developmental abnormalities in embryos
4 alterations in neuro-transmitter chemicals, resulting in behavioural abnormalities (he includes suicide as a behaviour disorder)
5 alterations in biochemical cycles
6 stress responses in exposed animals which, if prolonged, lead to loss of immune-system effectiveness
7 alterations in learning ability.

Becker makes the obvious point that more than one of these potential effects can occur in the same individual at the same time, each adding to the clinical condition. I go beyond Becker and say that radiation may be just one of a number of overload factors and these are cumulative also. The effects on a tired, stressed individual who is in poor nutritional balance and disturbed by unhappy life circumstances will be more severe. Such an individual is very vulnerable.

The original safety standard for radiation dosage of the microwave type was set at $100mW/cm^2$, which was based on the dose required to produce body heating. This was soon dropped to $10mW/cm^2$ but there it has stuck and the fallacy has arisen that this is a scientifically-judged figure.

Roger Coghill, research scientist, consultant and author of *Something in the Air*, tells me that current thinking is that electrical fields are probably more critical than magnetic flux, as was formerly thought. He recommends a safe level of 50 nanoTesla (nT).

Danger is certainly present beyond 250 nT. (A nanoTesla is about 10 volts per square metre). As Coghill points out, someone who spends most of his or her time in a typical home with levels of, say, 200–250 nanoTesla may actually receive more radiation in a year than someone who lives in a 'safe' house but is exposed to occasional doses of thousands or even tens of thousands of nanoTesla.[4]

WHAT YOU CAN DO

If you are concerned and would like to reduce your radiation exposure levels, you can help yourself quite a lot.

- Remove all unnecessary electrical devices from your bedroom, such as electric alarm clocks, radios and tea-makers.
- Get rid of electric blankets permanently. Forget about water beds; the electrical heater charges the water with persistent radiation.
- Avoid electrical equipment as much as possible and especially don't group such equipment near where someone sits or sleeps.
- You can have an EMF (electromotive force) demand switch fitted to your domestic supply which will turn off the mains at night but continue to supply the refrigerator and freezer (thus keeping you electricity-free for at least 8 hours a day.
- Stay at least 3 metres from your television screen and do not allow children to sit up close to it.
- If you have a mobile phone, buy a screen but make sure it's one which is effective. Some are not. Better still, get yourself a head set and keep the phone as far away from your brain as possible.
- If you use a computer or VDU, at home or at work, try to place it as far from your body as possible. Insist on a protective screen. Make sure you are not contaminated by someone else's equipment, either nearby or in the next room (soft x-rays and microwaves can travel through walls unhindered).
- Avoid precautionary or 'routine' medical and dental x-rays for check-up purposes. Women of childbearing years should

have x-rays only in the 10 days following menstruation. Though this is now in dispute, it is better to play safe. Allow no x-rays if you are trying to conceive. Children should never be x-rayed, except in a dire emergency.

Caution

Do not attempt any kind of screening or Faradic cage for protection, using meshes, metal plates or wires. *You could make things worse by inadvertently focusing or intensifying the electromagnetic fields.*

If you want to measure the ambient levels of radiation exposure, consider one of the simple field meters which are available on the Internet. Roger Coghill manufactures and sells a hand-held device called a *Field Mouse* which is designed to warn of levels over 200 nT or 25 V/m^2 (available from Coghill Research Laboratories).

SCHUMANN WAVES

One aspect of Earth's radiation which has only recently attracted attention as a health issue is the Schumann wave effect. The Earth's atmosphere, between the underside of the ionosphere and the surface (especially the salt oceans) forms what scientists call a resonating cavity magnetometer. Due to excitation by the Earth's own magnetism, sunspots and lightning storms, this cavity emits a transverse resonating waveband that we call Schumann waves, after the man who discovered them in the 1940s.

The actual frequency varies according to the height of the ionosphere and large-scale weather patterns, but is generally in the 8—10 Hertz range. I feel sure it is no coincidence that this frequency is virtually identical with that of the hippocampus of mammalian species.

How vital Schumann waves are to health was finally settled in the 1960s, when astronauts in space became inexplicably ill. Only when artificial Schumann waves were supplied in the rockets did humans feel healthy once more. What is worrying is that modern cities have very low levels of Schumann waves, as most of these waves are absorbed by the vast masses of concrete and metal buildings. The gradual lowering of the land water table has also added to the deficiency.

This must have severe and unavoidable health consequences for city dwellers. The loss of health-giving Schumann waves could be a contributory factor in 'sick building syndrome'. The time may come when we have to supply artificially-generated frequencies in office buildings and dwellings, to make them comfortable to live and work in. However, caution is needed. Simply supplying Schumann waves carries with it the very distinct danger of increased platelet aggregation (blood clotting); this in turn is a known risk factor in heart disease and strokes.

The key to this further complication seems to be 'plasma waves'. These are interactions between the Earth's magnetic field and mineral elements within the lithosphere (Earth's crust). The strength of the waves generated is very small, even by the standards of the Gaia fields, but what seems to be important is a resonance effect between the Earth's minerals and the same elements within living forms, especially the blood.[5]

At first sight it might appear that the oscillations from the electron shells of very many elements at once would simply create 'noise'. However, according to new theories, electron plasma waves have precise frequencies in the extremely low frequency (ELF) band (which, as I keep repeating, has a powerful biological impact). Trace minerals are present in very tiny amounts as constituents of vitamins, enzymes and hormones. Resonant frequencies from the Earth in these critical bands could have an enormous effect on these body chemical mediators.

If this is correct then we do seem to be, literally, children of Gaia.

THE GRIDS

As I reported in my book *The Allergy Handbook*, skilled dowsers have been able to find definite geometric grids which cross and re-cross the Earth's surface.[6] I refer here to the Curry Grid and the Hartman Net (both named after the doctors who discovered them). I am *not* here including ley lines. I have great confidence in the ability of certain dowsers and therefore accept the presence of these grids. Far too many people can find them. I myself have felt the rods kick when I was shown what to do by the great Kathe Bachler. However, I have always been troubled by the oddity of such geometric straightness or rigidity being imposed upon the natural organic order of things. I have since come across a model which may help us to gain more insight into this possibility.

It comes from an experiment carried out by pupils of Buckminster Fuller. A balloon submerged in coloured fluid and subject to vibration revealed geometric patterns where the dye had broken up into intersecting straight lines over the surface of the sphere. The classic icosahedron of the geodesic dome developed by Fuller came from this observation. It is truly a Gaia design. From this experiment it does seem that there are inherent energy formations on the surface of a sphere which follow straight lines (though not, of course, truly straight but bent to the shape of the sphere).

I was interested to learn that Polynesian sailors were able to navigate by following bands of 'light' under the ocean. Only a fool would now scoff at this idea. Perhaps the Australian aboriginal dream lines are also in some way connected with this surface grid phenomenon. I don't want to wander off into the realms of so-called Earth mysteries, ley lines, ancient temple sites and so on, though I can't exclude the possibility that they may be aspects of the same thing. I am merely making the point that there is a natural scientific validity in the existence of electromagnetic grids and patterns over the Earth's surface, and wish to imply the logical corollary that these must perforce have a health impact, for good or ill.

Such energy networks will also form a background of interference with the biological energy signals which can be detected by the equipment you have been reading about in this book.

RADIOACTIVITY

One of the most frightening and significant stressors of the human body arising in modern times is ionizing radiation pollution. It is appropriate to include this in a review of Gaia since, initially, radon seepage from rock such as granite or (more rarely) uranium was our only source of this deadly energy. Nowadays humanity produces such huge quantities of radioactivity that we are truly soiling our own nest and facing dire consequences.

It is an irony that radiation has saved the lives of many thousands of people, yet it is deadly to cells and all living tissue. Radiotherapy is now such a key feature of anti-cancer therapies that one may be forgiven for losing sight of the fact that it actually *causes* cancer. A wise thinker would recommend caution because of this paradox, rather than merely side-stepping it, as is normally the case. X-rays are so dangerous that mass radiography programmes had to be discontinued; it was concluded that screening for breast cancer was actually causing 5 per cent more cancers than it was detecting!

'Ionizing' radiation means that which harms us by causing alterations in the electrical status of the atoms and molecules of our body substances by wrecking the normal electrical bonding. The resulting charged particles are highly aggressive and can damage and even kill tissues when released. The extent of the damage depends on the dose, and herein is one of the major problems with this particular hazard, which is that doses are cumulative for life. That means all the radiation you have ever been faced with is added together in a running total. It does not 'wear off'.

In sufficient doses (by convention we speak as if it were a drug or medicine!) it causes radiation sickness, which is characterized by severe tissue damage, leading to loss of hair, loss of intestinal mucosa and severe disruption of the blood-forming tissues. The latter is particularly important, since it means the possibility of both anaemia and white cell (leukocyte) failure. Loss of viable leukocytes means the body is unable to defend itself from pathogens or cancerous invasion. Death is the usual outcome of severe radiation sickness. There is little that can be done to treat it. Those who survive often go on to develop cancer, leukaemia and, as we saw from Hiroshima and Nagasaki, genetic malformations.

Unfortunately, there is no 'standard' disease befalling an individual who has passed the safe quota for radiation. The effects show up simply as an increase in existing pathological conditions. This allows a great deal of official fudging about the true dangers of living near nuclear plants and 'hot' military installations.

By its very nature, the effects of chronic insidious exposure to ionizing radiation goes largely undetected, since we have no biological sensors with which to measure it. It is only when recognized polluters see fit to install monitoring equipment that we may know what is actually happening to our environment and the extent of the threat to our health. Spectacular melt-downs such as that at Chernobyl and the narrowly-averted Three Mile Island disaster may be the stuff we all fear; but there is good reason to believe that far more people are killed by radiation annually, without realizing it, than ever died in all the disasters put together. Again, official secrecy is keeping us in the dark, as if it were a government's right to deceive and dissemble to its people.

Yet leaks do occur. Such releases are not confined to nuclear reactors or weaponry, but take place at all stages of processing, from mining to the disposal of waste. Once in the environment, radioactive elements are concentrated in the food chain. We may be exposed to Caesium 137 in fish stocks up to 1,000 times the normal level; iodine sources are suspect since Chernobyl and, as we all know, strontium 90 has been a dangerous polluter of milk supplies since nuclear testing began in the 1960s.

The trouble is, most of these substances have a very long half-life. For strontium it is only 50 years, but plutonium 239 remains dangerously radioactive for 250,000 years.

Military Uses

While we are on the subject of plutonium, one aspect of nuclear weapons that is not well publicized is the EMP, or electromagnetic pulse phenomenon. An EMP is a very short, violent burst of electromagnetic energy that is produced when a nuclear weapon explodes in space. To quote Dr Robert D Becker again: 'If an EMP were produced by a nuclear explosion 100 miles above Kansas City, its energy would be so intense that it would shut off all electric-power systems, destroy all computers and magnetic disks or tape records, destroy the guidance systems of missiles and the computer and communications systems of military and commercial aircraft, and shut down all radio communications – *across the entire United States'* [his italics].[7]

In other words, it would bring the whole country to a halt.

Now the US military is trying to develop devices to produce EMPs without the need for a nuclear explosion. One can only hope that the fools who have sanctioned this idea are not the ones who control the likely use of such weapons. Otherwise, God help us all.

This is not a socio-political tract, I merely introduce the crude violence of the military mind to make the point that while officialdom is busily denying the very existence of any biological effects from ELF radiation, they have instructed the military to work out ways to use it to hurt people.

CRYSTALS

Finally, to sweeten the note, it is right to take a look at crystals in the context of Gaia. Thus we come back to holism instead of hazards. There is a large and flourishing healing movement using the properties of crystals to improve body energy.[8] The ordered structure of crystals has a constant, coherent and reproducible energy vibration. Crystals can be used to transmit, receive, amplify, modulate (transform) or ground (earth) energies. In fact, society as we know it could not exist without these properties of crystals; they are used in radio, television, computers and other electronic devices. The laser relies absolutely on the coherent intense light propagated by ruby.

Crystals can also store energy. If you hit a crystal with a mallet it will give off a brief flash of visible light; the so-called piezoelectric effect of rock crystal. Earth crust pressures do this on natural rock, as I explain in *The Allergy Handbook*, and this may be the source of many strange 'UFO' effects, especially in mountain zones, such as the Andes, where many strange lights are to be seen.[9]

If you consider that you are no more than flesh and blood, then you might reject the idea that crystals can affect you in any way. But if you have been following the main thread of this book and accept that we are a composite 'energy being' then you will readily understand it is quite obvious that crystals can influence our 'aura'. If you put a coherent crystalline structure in your body energetic field, it is bound to change it in some way; and if you are very sensitive you may even feel this.

Amethyst is known as a *receiver*. It was used in crystal radio sets. Popes and Bishops have traditionally worn amethyst rings to receive messages 'from above'. Rose quartz was also used in the days of crystal radio, but as a transmitter. Tourmaline is an amplifier, aquamarine a tuner and carnelian a grounder. Amazonite is said to open the higher psychic centres. I didn't know of this property when I once carried some in my pocket and had the strangest other-worldly sensations, until I realized what it was and removed it.

If you use a computer a great deal, you might like to introduce a large crystal next to it to absorb some of the radiation. Smoky quartz is said to be best. Try it if you believe this!

CHAPTER 11

HOW DOES YOUR GARDEN GROW?

Although not strictly a quantum or 'virtual' detection device in the sense of the methods introduced in the foregoing chapters, biological terrain assessment instruments come with a similar philosophy and standards of health care to the Vega, Mora, electro-dermal screening (EDS) and other derivative machines. Indeed, to date, the main doctors who use biological terrain assessment (BTA) analysis are those who already have one or more of the systems discussed.

Because it is not a 'mysterious' series of tests and relies largely on straightforward textbook principles of physiology (albeit much neglected in our drug-based medical culture), the BT assessment analysis should do a great deal to bridge the gap between scientific allopathic medicine and proven complementary therapy. This innovative approach has gained acceptance from doctors long before EAV, ayurvedic gem radiation or bioresonance. There is nothing here, other than the overall holism, to ruffle the feathers of hospital administrators and dyed-in-the-wool medical purists.

Nevertheless, you read it here first!

While a full understanding of biological terrain assessment would require considerable knowledge of biochemistry, physiology and clinical nutrition, the basic principles and the potential for practical use should not be beyond the grasp of any lay person, if we take it slowly.

HOW DOES YOUR GARDEN GROW?

First of all, what do we mean by the term 'biological terrain'? A good analogy is to compare it with growing food. Those who have lived on or near an arable farm, or have grown their own vegetables in the garden, will have had a wonderful opportunity to study plant care. It is obvious that there is more to it than scattering seeds and just waiting for something to happen. Nurturing plants successfully includes a knowledge of soil chemistry, meteorological conditions, nutrients and fertilizers, pest control (organic or not), adequate amounts of water and sunshine and a host of other factors which may or may not be consciously invoked but certainly play their part. The result is plants which are resistant to insects, moulds, bacteria and other pests. Kirlian photography of healthy natural foodstuffs shows a nice radiant 'aura', while weakened or improperly nourished plants show a feeble energy shell.

It is easy, then, to compare the human body tissues to the garden. Assessing biological terrain then means to be able to monitor and control the quality of the 'soil' so that we remain healthy despite the numerous attacks of invaders, such as bacteria, viruses, cancer cells and moulds. When the patient's body chemistry is balanced and maintained by a healthy, nutritious diet, with an adequate intake of vitamins and minerals, and sufficient exercise and rest, avoiding stressful situations, then the body – like the garden – can remain strong and healthy.

One of the our most important 'crops' is a vibrant and strong immune system. But just as a neglected crop fails to produce healthy food and becomes highly susceptible to diseases and tissue breakdown, if the human body is poorly fed and subjected to junk food, toxins, stress and inadequate maintenance, so it too will exhibit signs of ill-health. Unfortunately this 'unhealthy garden' state has become the norm, rather than the exception.

We call the garden our *milieu intérieur* or 'inner environment', a term coined by the great 19th-century French physician Claue Barnard. It is explained en passant to first-year medical students but then virtually disappears from view. No further thought is given to this elegant expression or the absolutely life-breathing physiology that it implies. Instead we get the spectacle of doctors trying to fight a disease such as cancer with the mentality of the Vietnam war. The approach is to decimate everything in sight, killing good and bad in the hope of annihilating the very last enemy cell, while turning the terrain into defoliated wasteland.

It didn't work on the larger scale and it violates common sense to suppose it will succeed on a biochemical scale.

BACKGROUND TO BT TESTING

In 1953 Professor Janos Kemeny, a biomathematician at the Polytechnic Institute in Budapest, demonstrated how we could monitor the *milieu intérieur* through three main parameters:

1 Mass or kinetic energy
2 Elasticity or sensibility factor
3 Viscosity or thermal factor.

In 1959 a young French hydrologist, Claude Vincent, further developed this concept and devised electrical testing which would give reasonably accurate estimates of the state of blood, urine and saliva, by means of three main 'soil' measurements,[1] as follows:

1 pH
2 Oxidation-reduction potential (Redox)
3 Resistivity (measured in Ohms).

Machines have since been developed which bring BTA testing into the marketplace in a way which is not merely affordable but is within the abilities of a typical busy medical practitioner in his own or her own surgery or clinic. The BTA S-2000 series, developed by Dr Robert C. Greenberg of Biological Technologies International, is at present the most advanced machine available and is currently in use in research departments at the University of Massachusetts, The Capital University of Integrated Medicine in Washington DC, and the World Health Organization.

The BTA 2000™ measures blood, urine and saliva in three ways:

1 Proton content (hydrogen ions, in effect)
2 Electron content
3 Mineral ion content.

The results are displayed in a schematic chart with four main quadrants, giving information about metals, fungus, cancer and general vitality. Extensive research and years of practical application have shown that this is a useful format for retrieving clinical information. Certain appearances allow a clinical estimation to be made almost at a glance.

EXTRA-CELLULAR FLUID

Our body cells and tissues are bathed in a fluid medium, which we call extra- (outside) cellular fluid or ECF. The fashion among doctors is to regard this as relatively unimportant – an incidental, just the 'stuff' which hangs around outside the cells, where it is considered the real action takes place.

This is to make a serious misjudgement. The extra-cellular fluid is the gateway to everything which happens within the cells. The ECF is akin to the soil in the garden; the cells are the crop. Our tissues are totally dependent on this fluid for the nutrients they receive and for the elimination of waste products. An unbalanced ECF will lead to a very poor crop indeed. Yet doctors continue to focus almost entirely on blood values, which they see as paramount. This fails to take into account that the blood is a highly buffered and protected fluid, where the chief organs such as heart, lungs, kidneys and liver work very hard to keep it up to standard, in terms of content.

Even when there is a general lack of an important nutrient, its level is maintained in the blood at all costs. For example it is little use measuring blood magnesium, because the body cannot tolerate even a tiny lowering of its presence without the heart ceasing to beat regularly. By the time blood magnesium falls, the body is in a serious negative equity situation, as it were.

The ECF feels the lack first, then the cells, then, *lastly*, the blood.

Isn't it strange, therefore, that a lab workup of a patient never includes routine measurements of the status of this vital nutrient fluid? That's why we commonly reach the situation where a patient goes through regular hospital screening and is told 'nothing is wrong,' when it is *obvious* that the patient looks ill, feels ill and is presenting with symptoms.

This is where BTA analysis can help. Valuable information

emerges which not only gives a new kind of diagnosis but also offers an intelligent breakthrough strategy for treatments. BT analysis tells us about the person's whole internal biochemical domain. If we treat this, instead of picking out only certain aspects of it, then we can bring the body back towards the optimum balance, with resulting benefit.

The Test

The patient fasts for 12–14 hours. He or she is told to avoid toothpaste, mouthwashes or lipstick, which could affect the chemistry of the mouth. An early-morning urine specimen is brought to the clinic, and immediately a venous blood sample is drawn and saliva collected. All three fluids are fed into the machine, which is basically a sensor device linked to a computer. There are nine scientific values determined and reported on. The practitioner assesses the print-out information and may then share it with the patient as a teaching guide.

The BT analysis testing procedure does not diagnose any specific pathology or disease states, although it will give strong pointers to certain afflictions, as you will see. Rather, its strength is that it serves as a series of important guide-posts that tremendously aid the overall management of the patient. We come back again to the dynamic energetic principle of health. The body is a non-linear domain and obeys the tumbling laws of chaos; it can only be intelligently assessed in these terms. It is *not* a collection of separate biochemical values. It is a nutrient sea or soup in which the life process takes place, endlessly evolving, endlessly varied.

Often the client has been a tough case and this may be the first time he or she begins to see why there have been so many 'failed' therapies. Bluntly, if nutrition and the *milieu intérieur* are faulty, nothing will truly succeed, neither good therapy nor bad.

INDIVIDUAL VALUES 1: PH

The pH of any fluid is basically a statement of the number of active hydrogen ions in the water solute. It is a logarithmic scale, from 0–14, though the outer values are largely theoretical. 7.0 is deemed to be the centre balance point; below this value denotes an acidic solution (excess hydrogen ions) and above this value denotes an alkali solution (relative lack of hydrogen ions). It is worth pointing out that a hydrogen ion is also called a *proton*, since it is minus its electron at this point.

Blood has a pH of around 7.4 and this is very critical (7.35—7.45). Any tendency to move away from this narrow range is adjusted by the body, which compensates by utilizing a chemical effect called *buffering*. Chiefly centred around the bicarbonate ion (an alkali ion), buffering is orchestrated by the kidneys and the lungs; specifically, by varying how much bicarbonate is retained by the kidneys and how much carbon dioxide (acid) the lungs breathe out.[2] The normal pH range of several other bodily fluids is shown here:

Bodily fluid	pH
Saliva	6.0—7.0
Gastric secretions	1.0—3.5 (very acidic)
Pancreatic secretions	8.0—8.3 (moderately alkaline)
Urine	4.5—8.0 (can be acidic or alkaline)
Bile	7.8 (slightly alkaline)

Latent Acidosis

Acids are produced by the body as a normal function of cellular metabolism. These acids greatly increase during times of stress (mental pollution), exercise and, of course, eating acid-forming foods. Even a simple sugar like glucose breaks down, in the presence of adequate oxygen, into carbon dioxide and water. The carbon dioxide dissolves in the water to make carbonic acid. Too much of this and the body has a problem, which is how to get rid of it.

The kidneys hold back more bicarbonate ions, to compensate for the acidity. When under pH stress, this means a big build-up of bicarbonate and trouble may ensue because saturation point will be reached eventually. If there is inadequate oxygen or lack of insulin, the body will divert foods into an alternative, so-called 'anaerobic' pathway (nothing to do with gym aerobics). This means the body will produce large quantities of non-volatile lactic acid and betahydroxybutyric acid, both of which are rapidly toxic in any quantities.

Another Factor in Therapy Resistance

So, one of the first insights that BTA analysis brings is that it shows us that *there is a latent acidosis accompanying almost all chronic disease*. Treating the condition without treating the acidosis is likely to lead to a recurrence. I am talking now about acidosis in the extra-cellular fluid or mesenchyme (Pischinger's matrix); the blood, naturally, is heavily buffered and it may remain within the basic range while the mesenchyme is loaded with non- volatile acids and is a long way off pH balance.[3] It makes no sense to use oxygen-activating therapy without addressing the total body acid/alkaline balance. The advantages of O_2 therapy are mopped up within minutes by the mesenchyme compensation.

The most common cause of acidosis is faulty nutrition. It begins with coffee and white bread and ends with sugar and alcohol; these have a synergistic effect. It is made worse by soft drinks, some of which (colas particularly) can be extremely acidic (phosphoric acid). These drinks also contain large amounts of sugar, which will draw both phosphorous and calcium from the bones, resulting in osteoporosis. It is shocking but hardly surprising that even young girls are now being found to have a degree of osteoporosis, due to excessive consumption of sugary soft drinks. Be warned!

Ironically, acid foods such as fruits are metabolized into bases (alkali) and actually help to reverse this destructive acidosis. The reader is warned to interpret published lists for so-called 'food combining diets' with care; Dr William Hay, who originally proposed food combining in the 19th century, was speaking of foods which are metabolized to acid or alkaline ash. It makes no difference which the food is *before* you eat it; you must categorize it by what it becomes when metabolized.

Getting Back to Alkaline

You can produce a quick result, but I must emphasize that it is in no sense a proper remedy or 'cure', by taking alkali salts. Sodium bicarbonate enjoys a historical place, since people have evidently found it helps. But the optimum formula that we call alkali salts is a mixture of two parts sodium bicarbonate to one part potassium bicarbonate. Take 1–2 teaspoons of this formula in half a tumbler of water. Aim for a morning urine pH of 6.5–7.0.

Proper medication would consist of metabolic assistance in the form of homeopathic remedies to support the proper chemical pathways, particularly the Kreb's cycle for aerobic processing of energy foodstuffs. Liver, pancreas and kidney drainage are also indicated.

A long-term and definitive strategy comes from dietary modification. Certain foods are alkaline-forming and, surprise surprise, these are the ones usually recommended for health and vitality – chiefly fruit, nuts, vegetables and beans.

INDIVIDUAL VALUES 2: REDOX

One of the hot topics in medicine at present is oxidative stress, meaning tissue damage and ageing caused by attack from highly active chemicals or pollutants. Oxygen itself is quite toxic in excess, but what is meant here is chemical oxidation – that is, the stripping of electrons from the cells (the donating of electrons is called reduction). This type of tissue damage is a known risk factor in developing cancer, and also in the ageing process.[4]

So much has been written in the last two decades about oxidation and reduction (redox potential) that it has practically become a science in its own right. Redox potential is basically a way of stating the chemical reactivity of a substance or fluid and is explained as follows:

All life is composed of molecules which have a greater or lesser degree of complexity. Molecules are made up of two or more tiny particles called *atoms*. Some larger molecules have many thousands of atoms but are still inconceivably small. Atoms have a charged nucleus, or centre, which contains protons and neutrons. Around these whirl electrons, though the quantum researchers have been at this model and say that electrons may only be standing waves.

Keeping to the simple view, electrons are negatively charged and are balanced by protons at the centre, which are positively charged, keeping the whole electrically neutral. Neutrons, as their name implies, are neither positive nor negative, so it doesn't matter how many there are. Atoms with different numbers of neutrons are called isotopes, but we shall not need this term here.

In the process of a chemical reaction, it is the electrons which migrate from one atom to another and so bind them into molecules. Redox potential is nothing more than a quantitative measurement of how fiercely the electrons want to seize each other's domain. Where the overall tendency is to give up electrons, we call it reduction. Where electrons are needed, this is an oxidizing system.[5]

Redox potential (usually labelled E) is measured in the electrical value of milli-volts (mV). Negative values mean a tendency to oxidize; positive values mean a tendency to reduce.

Redox potential gives us information about two very important body processes:

1 creating high-cellular energy in the form of ATP (adenosine tri-phosphate), which is like petrol at the cellular level and drives the processes within the cell.
2 the ability to oxidize or burn up pollutants, xenobiotics and some species of micro-organisms; rather like a rubbish bonfire.

Thus it will be readily appreciated that if the body runs out of cellular fuel, or loses its ability to eliminate chemical waste, we get big health problems. In fact we would get a state very like chronic fatigue syndrome or ME, where the main symptom is lack of energy and the main contributory factor is toxic overload.

When a life-sustaining fluid like blood is loaded with electrons (and therefore has a high negative E value), the potential for potent energizing and potent life-giving chemical reactions is proportionately high. If it should become positive in E value, it has spent all of its kinetic energy and is low in potential energy.

Actually, in biological systems, the expression E is replaced by the symbol rH_2, which has to do with the way it is measured (force of hydrogen [H_2] as it appears at the cathode).

The rH_2 measurement provides a quick index to the body's biochemical make-up. In today's world, where oxidative stress comes from so many sources such as traffic fumes, plastics, synthetics, food additives, air pollution and medicinal products, the ability to quickly and accurately assess the extent of the damage along these grounds is a godsend to the holistic practitioner who is concerned with such issues.

INDIVIDUAL VALUES 3: RESISTIVITY

This is probably the easiest of the three values to understand. It means the electrical conductivity of the tissues, which in turn is determined by their mineral content.[6] Minerals are vital to the proper nutrient status of the body, functioning as co-enzymes in vital chemical pathways, co-vitamins, for example magnesium and zinc with B_6, and of course in tissue repair.

A high resistivity of the fluid samples of BTA analysis would therefore imply a loss of nutrient vitality and big problems for the patient.

It has long been a contention of mine, shared by an increasing number of practitioners, that no healing process works well or may not work at all if the patient has inadequate nutritional levels. However, this is not a situation where 'more is better'. There are optimum levels for all substances in the healthy body. If excess mineral salts are not removed when required they may build up in the body where they are not wanted. In other words, minerals can become toxic in excess. A simple example should suffice: calcium is needed in optimum quantities in bone, but where it is not required, such as in arteries, around joints and in the cerebral tissue, it forms calcified deposits and these accelerate ageing.

Below are listed the main normal values for these measurements in healthy humans.[7] Originally these were values for fit athletes but, as a standard to aim for in routine health care, these former ideal levels have been relinquished in favour of more ordinary and attainable values.

OPTIMAL VALUES

	pH	Redox	Resistivity
Blood	7.30–7.35	21.5–23.5	190–210
Saliva	6.50–6.75	21.5–23.51	80–220
Urine	6.50–6.80	22.5–24.5	30–45

Derived Values

The BTA 2000™ incorporates software which includes an estimate of 'biological age' or tissue potency. As in Chapter 5, I repeat that this has *no connection* with calendar age. The latter is used only as a reference. BTA values which are significantly higher than the average for the patient's actual age would give a raised biological age. As treatment progresses, biological age may fall, whereas if calender age were included as one of the variables, this would of course remain static, and of no value as an indicator of improvement.

The higher the biological age, the more tissue stress and the greater the reduction in a person's powers of recovery. This is shown even more explicitly in the bar graph called the 'cellular defence index'. If this value falls too far out of range, it calls into question whether the patient's tissues really do have sufficient powers of recovery to reverse the deterioration trend.

Casebook: Male, 43 Years

This is a case from the files of Dr Jeffrey Klass of Branford, Connecticut.[8] A patient reported to him complaining of obesity and chronic fatigue. He had tried numerous diets and exercise programmes but had got nowhere.

The first BT analysis showed him to be a fast oxidizer, with a blood pH of less than 7.45 (7.37 actual). This meant he was metabolically unsuited to carbohydrates, confirmed by a raised salivary pH of 7.18. Dr Klass put him on a low carbohydrate diet, with plenty of protein, fat and cooked vegetables, together with pancreatic enzyme supplementation to aid digestion and metabolism.

Male, 43 Years: First BT Analysis Values

	pH	Redox	Resistivity
Blood	7.37	28.0	262
Saliva	7.18	29.9	347
Urine	5.58	21.9	104

The raised urine pH was indicative of mild kidney overload. The picture also revealed high oxidative stress in blood and saliva (28.0 and 29.9 respectively). The very high values for resistivity are classic for a demineralized patient. His biological age was 67.

The correct regimen, therefore, included plenty of nutrient minerals, especially zinc, potassium and magnesium, along with a good vitamin complex. Klass also prescribed herbal detox formula and liver, kidney and lymphatic formulas.

One month later, the repeat BT analysis showed values which were in several respects higher:

Male, 43 Years: Second BT Analysis Values

	pH	Redox	Resistivity
Blood	7.4	27.9	322
Saliva	7.26	30.1	428
Urine	5.56	22.2	106

The salivary pH was even worse, reconfirming poor carbohydrate metabolism. Oxidative stress was worse in the saliva also, pointing to deterioration in liver or lymphatics. Mineralization was worse. What had gone wrong?

It emerged that the patient had not followed his diet and had taken his supplements only fitfully. Duly chagrined, the patient promised to comply. Klass took the opportunity to add an antioxidant.

One month later the picture was dramatically improved:

Male, 43 Years: Third BT Analysis Values

	pH	Redox	Resistivity
Blood	7.39	25.6	187
Saliva	6.86	27.5	650
Urine	5.42	21.2	55

Blood pH had not improved but salivary pH had decreased, showing an increased ability to metabolize carbohydrates. Urinary pH showed that the kidneys were better able to eliminate the acidosis. Oxidative stress was improved across the boards. This shows that the body was able to produce more ATP (adenosine tri-phosphate) and utilize it more fully. Liver and lymphatic function had greatly improved.

The resistivity was now in the optimum range, showing that the supplement formulas were beginning to bite.

The clinical picture? The patient had lost 20 pounds, had much more energy and was delighted.

WHAT YOU CAN DO

Until BT analysis becomes more widely available to guide therapeutic regimes, you can benefit from some common-sense knowledge derived from this new technology. A number of changes in diet and lifestyle are complementary and can produce benefits to the 'soil' in numerous ways.

Reducing Oxidative Stress

1   Take antioxidant formula (vitamins A, C, E, zinc and selenium), plus magnesium and glutathione.
2   Eliminate as much chemical pollution from your home and workplace as possible.
3   Reduce or eliminate tea, coffee and alcohol.
4   Take co-enzyme formula and n-acetyl-carnitine, to aid cellular metabolism.
5   Eliminate or reduce exposure to electromagnetic and ionizing radiation.

Reducing Acidosis

6   Change your diet to exclude acid foods and increase the alkaline foods. Less meat, dairy, grains and eggs and more fruit, vegetables, beans and nuts.

7   Drink plenty of pure water to assist kidney elimination.

8   Reduce stress, fatigue, sugar and social poisons (alcohol, tobacco, so-called 'recreational' drugs).

9   Consider a liver cleanse (see page 82) and suitable homeopathic complexes to support liver, lymphatics and kidneys.

10   Make use of reflexology, aromatherapy, shiatsu and other soothing therapies.

Improving Resistivity (Mineralization)

11 Take a proper mineral supplementation formula. Avoid high doses, as minerals can compete with each other for absorption.

12 Take enough exercise and relaxation.

13 Use an oral chelation formula (check proprietary brands) to help eliminate heavy metal toxicity.

14 Consider dental amalgams as a source of metal overload (see Chapter 12).

15 Reduce food allergies and re-colonize the gut with probiotic formulas (L acidophilus and Bifidobacteria), to aid normal absorption.

In general, all the steps I refer to as my ortho-immune therapy apply to improving biological terrain: eliminating stress foods (junk items and those foods you personally tolerate poorly), taking nutrient supplements, undertaking a chemical clean-up, cleansing your system of parasites and cleaning up your life!

Complex homeopathy, specifically aimed at the matrix or mesenchyme therapy, is the science of cleansing and nurturing the inner garden. All 'drainage' remedies have cleansing and support properties. Nosode therapy (see page 118) is also about enriching the soil and eliminating pests.

CHAPTER 12

WEIRD OR WHAT?

Right at the start of the 20th century, the biggest single risk factor for death due to heart disease was tooth and jaw infections. Numerous pathology specimens in medical school museums, showing sub-acute bacterial endocarditis, cavernous sinus thrombosis and brain abscesses, testify to just how precarious life could be in the age before antibiotics (and also what we may be facing again if we go on abusing them foolishly). A single unhealthy tooth could lead to an early grave. Now, at the very end of the century, what do you suppose is among the biggest predictors of death due to heart disease?

Teeth. Well, more exactly, gum disease. This one risk factor has recently been shown to be just as important as smoking, obesity, blood pressure or an unfortunate family history in determining whether you or I will die before we should.[1] This seems very new and startling. Yet it has been talked about by EAV practitioners for decades and by switched-on dentists like Weston Price for even longer than that. Why is what goes on in your mouth so dangerous?

Well, as my holistic dentist friend John Roberts, secretary of the British chapter of the International Academy of Oral Medicine and Toxicology, points out, teeth sockets are a royal highway for disease pathogens leading straight into your bones. If we were to piece together all the patches of infection that a dentist sees in a typical mouth, he tells me it would be the equivalent of an ulcer eating away at half the back of your hand. Would you stand for that? Of course not, you say. But that's exactly what most of us are doing – we just don't see it in our jaw bones.

A tooth abscess is really just another kind of osteomyelitis – that is, bacterial bone infection. We take the condition of our teeth far too lightly. No-one in his or her right mind would allow a hole to be drilled into a femur or other bone and have it left draining to the outside world; serious infectious complications would be bound to ensue. Yet that is what we do with our teeth; some people live with what is virtually an open wound.

The position is not helped by techniques such as the crowning of teeth. It may make them appear cosmetically attractive on the outside. But often these metal or plastic caps do nothing more than cover and hide a seat of purulent infection, waiting to explode at some time in the future when the body's defences are compromised.

In an address on 'The Role of Sepsis and Antisepsis in Medicine' to the Faculty of Medicine at McGill University, Montreal, in 1910, Dr William Hunter baited his colleagues by saying, 'Knowing as we do the pathogenic qualities of staphylococci and streptococci, we have not the slightest excuse for allowing the mouth, so easily accessible to local measures, to remain the chief seat and a veritable hotbed for their development and propagation; on the contrary, it is a severe reflection on our profession if we allow it.'[2]

Elsewhere, in a piece in the *Lancet*, the enlightened Hunter referred to gold fillings, gold caps, gold bridges, gold crowns and fixed dentures built in, on and around diseased teeth as 'a veritable *mausoleum* of gold'. I feel sure he chose the word advisedly.

BACK PRESSURE

The late Patrick Stortebecker, Professor of Neurology at the Karolinska Institute in Stockholm, Sweden, carried out a series of experiments in the 1960s which I consider highly illuminating. The results were also rather scary.

Stortebecker injected tooth bone margins under pressure with radio-opaque dyes and then took x-rays of the skull. What he showed was that most head veins do not have valve control and therefore blood could travel backwards into the cranium; his radio-opaque dye appeared all over the head, far away from the tooth in which was injected. Obviously this effect will take place in life; all it needs is for a change of pressure gradient, which is what happens every time you sneeze or strain at stool. This was a controlled hygienic experiment, but if the tooth in question should happen to be infected, the results could be very adverse indeed. Bacterial toxic matter could be propelled into the cranium and there set up an unwanted focus of infection right inside the skull.[3] Stortebecker himself mentioned the obvious risk of cavernous sinus thrombosis and suppuration. This was once a killer condition. The cavernous sinus is a large vein reservoir at the base of the brain, and if it should clot and become filled with purulent matter, widespread meningitis and brain abscesses were the almost inevitable result. Many fatal tragedies from nose picking and spot scratching took place in former times; those of us old enough may remember that parents tended to frown on this behaviour and we were slapped. Now you know there was a scientific reason for the almost universal injunction against spot scratching.

We no longer see this morbid condition in Western medicine, thankfully. But it lurks just beyond view, always a threat from dental infections, averted simply by the use of antibiotics. If we should lose the availability of an effective non-toxic antibiotic, as seems very probable the way they are being over-prescribed and pushed by drug companies, then worrying times will return.

But that's not all. Stortebecker had another disease model which I find very persuasive. He considers that what he found is the principal factor in the pathogenesis of multiple sclerosis.[4] Through extensive research he was able to show that most plaques of nerve de-myelination (the unmistakable sign of MS) were located around blood vessels. No-one else had noticed this important fact before. Stortebecker speculated that the back-pressure on veins had shunted toxic matter into the brain tissues, where it set up foci of inflammation and myelin loss. What was particularly convincing was that MS cases with optic neuritis (leading to blindness) generally had bad teeth and inflammation plaques in the brain; whereas those who had leg weakness or paralysis, with de-myelination plaques in the spinal cord, had pelvic or other lower-body disease foci. EAV folk find that the pelvic organs in particular hide a great deal of smouldering pathology. I myself have started to speak of a woman's 'angry pelvis', it is so common and so much undermines a woman's well-being.

Unfortunately, Stortebecker is gone. Apart from a handful of us, his work is ignored and it is very difficult to interest anyone in the medical establishment. Dentists don't even want to think about it. Doctors say it's a dental problem and nothing to do with them. Thus we have here another sad example of how specialization can make medicine ineffective. But the possibility that this hypothesis is sound requires that it be investigated scientifically, with adequate funding and proper protocol.

Just don't hold your breath.

TOXIC DENTISTRY

It is not really stretching the human mind too far to suggest that most dentistry is, by its nature, quite toxic. Modern methods rely heavily on materials such as metals, plastics and polymers, ceramics and prosthetic structures of many kinds. Unfortunately, EAV practitioners are discovering that most of this foreign material is stressful to the body. It can be a considerable drain on the immune system and therefore a major contributory cause of fatigue and chronic ill-health. In this new context we can only urge people even more emphatically to try to prevent dental problems from starting up. Good diet and adequate teeth hygiene may, even in this day of antibiotics, still be a key life-saver.

I do not exaggerate.

COOKED TEETH

Recent research by Ralph Turk and Fritz Kronner in Germany has shown that even the act of drilling a tooth causes severe energy disturbance.[5] Turk describes the modern dental turbine rotor as a sort of time-bomb, and that its damaging intensity has been completely missed by the vast majority of dentists. There are many likely reasons for this damage, not least being the fact that, despite water cooling, the temperature of the dentine rises by as much as 10 degrees after just a few *seconds* of drilling. In biological terms this is cooking the tooth. This denaturation obviously destroys the viability of the tooth and its ability to resist bacterial invasion. From over 6,000 cases studied it was uniformly seen that, as soon as a tooth was visited by a high-speed drill, focal osteitis trouble began in connection with that tooth within 2 years.

It is possible to reduce the damage by taking sensible anti-tox procedures before, during and after a dental programme. EAV tests show that this at least minimizes the impact of high-tech dentistry. Such elementary measures would include taking vitamin C, charcoal (to absorb toxins), homeopathic support and immune drainage remedies such as Heel's lymphomyosot or Pascoe's Pascotox (Chapter 7 covers complex homeopathy).

MERCURY

Then there is the mercury story. Just over a decade ago, most of us were still to be convinced of the problem of biological intoxication with mercury. Official bodies such as the British and American Dental Associations deny it still.

As I said in my last book, gram for gram, mercury is one of the most toxic substances known to humanity, and it is arguably the most serious environmental pollutant we are creating for ourselves. Unfortunately mercury, especially in the methyl or chloride forms which have great biological penetration, has a special affinity for brain tissue. Most people know that the expression 'mad as a hatter' comes from the fact that twitching and dementia were once common among hat manufacturers and were due to poisoning with the mercuric nitrate used for curing felt hat bands.

The first health scare of modern times was the discovery that in the 1950s children who were dying of pink disease were being poisoned by mercury in 'teething powders'. Then, in 1953, the inhabitants of the Japanese fishing port of Minamata began to fall ill with a mysterious illness which caused twitching, mental confusion, difficulty in speaking and eventually paralysis. Autopsy showed considerable brain damage and the agent was discovered to be mercury. A nearby factory was dumping mercuric waste into the bay, which contaminated the fish stocks. It was concentrated in the food chain and reached deadly levels before being eaten by humans.

Despite all this, the dental profession continues to insist mercury is somehow non-toxic when you put it in your mouth! There is considerable hypocrisy about this, however; the instructions to dentists for handling mercury leave no doubt that it is harmful to dentists – even though it is supposed to be safe for patients. Advice to the profession includes storing it under water, not touching it by hand, providing adequate air extraction to eliminate the toxic vapour, and so on. Generally it is illegal for dentists to allow fluids contaminated by mercury to be sent into the sewage system. Filters or extractors are required.

The official argument was once that mercury remains firmly in the teeth and cannot spread to other tissues. Then in 1989 a team of doctors in Calgary, Canada, under Drs Hahn and Vimy, proved that the truth was very different. Using radioactive mercury and placing fillings in the teeth of sheep, they were able to show that mercury from fillings spreads all over a mammalian body *within hours*. The official line then switched to saying that there was no proven connection between mercury poisoning from amalgams and any known disease. This is specious and dishonest. It is not the public's job to prove there is a danger from mercury; it is the manufacturer's responsibility to show that it is safe. There is no prospect of this being possible.

The reason that the precipitating role of amalgams in disease processes is being missed is that doctors do not ask the right question: have you ever visited your primary care physician with a complaint and been asked 'Have you recently had any dental treatment?' Naturally, not. If doctors did check this important point they would be shocked at how often the answer would be yes.

What EAV doctors have been finding for years is that heavy metal overloads are a common cause of pathology and, not surprisingly, mercury is the godfather of all. Time and again mercury fillings are at the head of what I described in Chapter 8 as Causal Chains. However, this is not confined to mercury. Poisoning from other metals can occur. Sometimes the question is one of sensitivity, rather than poisoning.

We must accept what Nature tells us, and on testing a male patient with the Acupro I found that the biggest Indicator Drop pointed to danger from a gold-filled tooth and *not* the more obvious opposing amalgam. Scanning the dental nosode list showed that this patient was unusual in reacting to gold. I prescribed a homeopathic detoxification treatment and, next day, the gold filling fell out. Clearly it was rejected by the body, once given a little energetic help. The bemused patient preferred to believe it was 'just a coincidence', even though the tooth had remained in place for almost 20 years.

GALVANIC FIELDS AND ENERGETIC DISTURBANCE

Slightly more bizarre is the phenomenon of electrical fields around certain teeth and the effects these produce. I remember well the first time I saw Hal Huggin's slides of teeth cut open to show the scorch marks, where electrical current had been running for many years. Teeth can work like little batteries. This is quite logical: there are two or more metals and a saltwater fluid medium (saliva). This is how Allessandro Volta's original batteries were made; the battery of your motorcar is essentially the same thing.

The trouble starts from the fact that electrical currents actually leach the mercury out of the teeth, because of an effect called electrolysis. This is why patients sometimes complain of a constant metallic taste in the mouth, made worse by hot fluids and salty food (more electrolysis). If that isn't scary enough, then the reader should know that electrolysis is capable of releasing deadly mercury vapour. This goes straight to the brain tissue where it is highly invasive and toxic.

But the problem is even more complicated. The currents generated by amalgams can be quite considerable, and these are being formed very close to brain tissue, which operates at far lower potentials (a few millivolts). I have seen momentary spikes of up to 1 volt when testing teeth for the battery effect; this is enough to light a small torch battery. Remember the brain is really only a few millimetres from the jaw bone where the roots of the teeth lie, just the other side of the thin cranial bone and the meninges. Thus there is potential for mental dysfunction and this is often found in clinical practice, if the appropriate questions are asked.

Casebook: Female, 44 Years

The patient had suffered from Meniere's disease: vertigo and vomiting, with intermittent staggering (sailor's gait). She could not think clearly any more, had trouble with her memory, could not see clearly – lines appeared not straight. This was accompanied by pain in the nape of the neck. She was unable to continue working, due to the severity of these symptoms. Her attending physicians could find no clinical explanation and the patient was told it was all in her head (in a way this was true!). Finally, a brain tumour was suspected and tests were required to exclude this grim possibility.

The patient's luck eventually turned and an ENT surgeon referred her to Dr Helmut Raue, an EAV specialist who understands biological dentistry, as this new speciality is called. He measured her teeth galvanically and found 215 microamperes of current between a gold filling and a nearby amalgam. One week after having the amalgam removed, all pain had disappeared and the patient's balance had returned to normal. The patient admitted then that she had had suicidal thoughts because of the excruciating pain and baffling dizziness.[6]

The reason that not enough of these cases are being diagnosed and the true picture not emerging is that patients do not, usually, consult their dentist with symptoms such as headache, facial neuralgia, dizziness, sleep disorders and digestive disturbance (just to give a few examples).

ENERGETIC FIELDS

EAV practitioners are finding teeth foci as a common cause of energetic disturbance. The problem is immensely more complicated than it at first might seem. Several key acupuncture meridians cross the line of the teeth as they pass over the face. An abscess or 'transmitting focus' can actually create pathological results anywhere along the line of that meridian. These are further connected with secondary organs and sites. Thus problems with a front incisor tooth may impact on the kidneys, since this meridian passes through the incisors. But the kidneys, in turn, are related to the knee joints. If I see a patient with incisor problems or a bridge in this location I can surprise him or her by asking about the arthritis of the knees.

Sometimes the consequences of these interconnections are very surprising and virtually beggar explanation but should make us very wary indeed about the effects of dentistry.

Casebook: Female, 33 Years

A dentist had prepared a new crown tooth prosthesis, the type with a post of nickel which fits in a hole drilled down the centre of the tooth to give support. As the dentist offered the post to its new location on the right upper jaw, the woman let out a squeal: she'd gone immediately blind in that eye! The dentist removed the tooth and she could see again. He offered it back and she went blind again. This was repeated several times until both were quite sure of what they were observing.

She refused the crown and had the tooth removed instead.

What this striking case example of what we might call 'virtual dentistry' tells us is that energetic fields in the mouth are important to brain function. This was an *instant* reaction; there was no way it could depend on any chemical manifestation, even metal toxicity. Allergies to nickel do occur, though this metal is far less poisonous than mercury. But any such allergy would take a little time to develop. The striking part of the story is the *instant* loss of vision, which indicates clearly neurological dysfunction along the optical pathways due to a field disturbance, probably at the quantum or information level.

It also makes vividly clear what risks we take when we allow metal into our mouths. The resulting disturbance of the body's energy field can have unpredictable and very serious consequences. *I try to imagine in this case what would have happened if the woman had not lost her vision immediately but had gone blind over the subsequent few weeks.* Almost certainly the correct cause would never have been diagnosed. She may have ended up with harmful and unnecessary interventions which would fail because they were not aimed at correcting the real problem. It could even have made the situation worse.

ENERGETIC MERIDIAN RELATIONS WITH TEETH

Figure 11 shows the main teeth relations with acupuncture meridians. There are charts published which give a great deal of detail about these biological dental inter-relationships, but I have tried to simplify this down to the general picture for the reader. It is both interesting and enlightening to see these connections which were revealed for the first time through EAV.

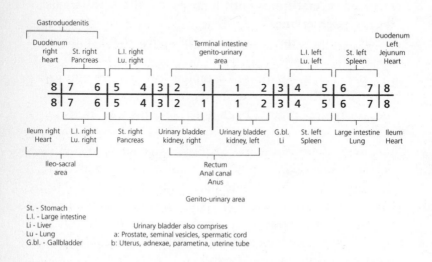

NICO: WHAT'S IN A NAME?

NICO is an EAV disease. By that I mean only EAV people would usually detect this curious type of pathology. It's a dental problem and has only come to light recently as a result of dentists doing their own EAV testing, though in fairness other good dentists do come across it.

NICO is an abbreviation of neuralgia-inducing cavitational osteonecrosis. I will explain. First, let me remind you that disease under the roots of teeth is a kind of bone inflammation, hence the term 'osteitis'. Osteonecrosis means the bone has died or lost its viability as a result; it is softened and eaten away, like rot in an apple. Neuralgia-inducing means that it has been postulated as a potent cause of neuralgia of the face, particularly that vicious kind known as trigeminal neuralgia. The trigeminal nerve (5th cranial nerve, emerging at the ear) is largely sensory and supplies the face, jaws and teeth. A phenomenon known as referred pain means that trouble anywhere within the nerve net can be felt at other places supplied by the same nerves. Thus NICO is a factor to consider in migraine or any kind of atypical headache. It is worth pointing out that the jaws are the only major bony tissue with important sensory nerve endings.

The 'cavitational' part of the name simply means some kind of cyst or space in the jaw bone, not necessary infected or inflammatory. Quite common is a fatty osteitis, where an old focus of inflammation has finally settled down and turned into a fatty cyst. There may be blood or chocolate matter in the cavity. But the important point which knowledgeable dentists are making is that this is not really an inflammatory process but tissue destruction caused by insidious loss of blood supply. In this respect it is more like other textbook bone diseases, where destruction comes from impaired blood and nutritional supply, which in 1915 US dentist G. V. Black described as progressive 'death of bone, cell by cell'.[7]

NICO is not rare. In one population study it was found in 1 in every 4,900 adults. This makes NICO by far the most common osteonecrotic bone disease; once again, specialization means that doctors are not talking to dentists as they should. NICO has been seen in people aged 18–94, but typically affects people in the 35–65 age range. An individual may have more than one focus of this disease process. It is hard to avoid the conclusion that it is the result of poor dental hygiene and maintenance; in other words, the consequence of burnt-out chronic infective foci.

Whatever the primary cause, bone cavities are open to subsequent bacterial invasions. Because the underlying process is caused by lack of oxygen these are likely to be anaerobic bacteria which release dangerous toxins and may in our present view be pre-malignant. Substances such as mercaptan and thioether, which are found regularly in dental foci by electro-dermal screening (EDS), are known carcinogens. It is unfortunate that NICO is usually not visible on x-ray. Many cases are missed even by experienced diagnosticians, since 35–50 per cent of bone loss is necessary before changes become radiographically evident. This is where EAV and virtual dentistry come in. I know dentists who are bold enough, and trust good EAV practitioners sufficiently, to drill into bone at the site indicated as a reading focus. It is very satisfying to both parties when the cortex is breached and a cavity filled with biological sludge makes its presence known.

Once diagnosed, treatment is currently by curettage of the site, sweeping away all the dead and softened bone, and maybe the first millimetre or so of healthy bone, in the hope that new, good bone will form. Coral granules may be used to pack the hole and encourage re-calcification of bone tissue. In about a third of cases this radical treatment fails and may even make the problem worse, but according to one writer only about 10 per cent of patients feel that the process wasn't worthwhile. Curettage is rather heroic and I have no doubt that in future something a little less aggressive will be the rule. While NICO is chiefly the domain of holistic dentists, such 'commando cures' are rather untypical of holism in general.

ROOT CANAL FILLINGS

Here is a topic where conventional medicine, decades ago, stood right where alternative innovative dentists stand today. The story is a fascinating one and begins in the first decade of this century with one Dr Billings. His research, published in 1914, showed that 95 per cent of all focal infections in the body came from the teeth and tonsils. Billing's work, in turn, was found by Weston Price, a leading dentist of his day. Price was an advocate of a healthy natural lifestyle and keynote nutrition; in every way he was a great thinker and a pioneer of values that we cherish today.

Price had a woman patient for whom he had done a root canal filling. She subsequently developed bad arthritis; it was so severe that she had become bedridden most of the time and her hands were so badly swollen she could barely feed herself. Price was honest enough to ask the question that no dentist cares to ask: could he have made her ill systemically by propagating generalized infection, as Billings had shown? He removed the root-canal-filled tooth, carefully and aseptically, to see what would happen. The woman promptly recovered.

From this case forward Price became very interested in the problem of root canal fillings. He had considerable success in helping patients, and published his results widely. There are copious papers by him in the medical and dental literature, most of it from the early 1920s. It is important to recognize that Price was a leading conventional dentist of the day. His views were listened to and, for a time, it became the fashion among doctors to recommend extracting teeth with root canal fillings as a cure for arthritis.

In fact this progressed to widespread tooth extractions, root canals or not, which was not what Price originally taught. Unfortunately, many cases did not recover as expected. The patient not only continued to suffer the arthritis but was now without any teeth. The approach became unpopular and was eventually discontinued. As a result, Price's views were discredited and lost sight of. It was one of those cases where the pendulum swung too far in a particular direction. Price was right, of course, but there needed to be some way of choosing patients who would benefit from removing root canal fillings.

Voll gave us the means. It is now a common aspect of EDS diagnosis to consider the safety and validity of root canal fillings.

They may not be a problem. If the person is fit and strong, with a good immune system, the situation can continue unchanged for many years. But if at some time in the future he or she undergoes too much stress or suffers from a major illness, resistance may be compromised and the dangers of root canals become manifest and dangerous.

The problem is that, although root canal work looks fine on x-ray and it might appear that there is a perfect occlusion of the former root canal down the heart of the tooth, microscopic examination reveals a different story. Tooth dentine, which is hard and screeches like rock when the dentist attacks it with his drill, is really composed of numerous tiny tubules. It is said there are 3 miles of end-to-end tubules in every tooth; they are supposed to conduct nutrients to keep the tooth alive and healthy. When bacteria gain access to the tooth, they lurk in these tubules. Filling the root canal does not flush the pathogens out of this domain. In fact the bacteria are then trapped in a closed-off space and inevitably cause trouble.

Pathogens have to go somewhere when they multiply. They can migrate through what are called lateral tubules and escape into the periodontal membrane and subsequently into the bony tissue of the jaw. From there they migrate around the body. As biological dentist and author of *Root Canal Cover Up*[8] George Meinig puts it:

These bacteria are kind of like people, if they get to like Seattle or Reno or someplace they decide that's where they are going to have their home. Well, the bacteria travelling round the body, they may get to the liver, the kidneys or the heart or eyes or some other tissue and they set up an infection in that area. This is why the degenerative diseases occur from the teeth.[9]

TRANSMITTING TEETH

Now we come to the part that is definitely weird, hence the title of this chapter. Everything so far is at least logical, if rather unnerving. It makes sense. From here it makes no real sense, except in the insubstantial quantum domain or, as we would once have said, 'the etheric'. What Weston Price did in the 1920s was to take infected and pathogenic root-canal-filled teeth and surgically stitch them into rabbits for observation. This is an example of one of those experimental situations like Benjamin Franklin sending his kite up into a thunderstorm: a mixture of perverse genius and intuition that leads to some important scientific insight.

What Weston Price found was that the rabbits became ill with the same diseases as the patients, or if not exactly the same diseases, then the same organ was attacked in some way. If the human had nephritis (cured after tooth extraction), then the rabbit got nephritis; if the human had heart disease, cancer or arthritis, that was what the rabbit got. Eye problems were particularly striking; if the human had only mild eye trouble, the rabbit would react so severely as to go blind in two or three days.

The only real conclusion is that the tooth carried some message of disease using an unknown code. Whether it was a quantum field factor or some other means of information transference is simply not known. You would think this absolutely fascinating series of experiments would have scientists racing to investigate the significance of what Price found. Instead, his work was promptly forgotten for over 50 years. So much for the progress of scientific thought.

WHAT YOU CAN DO

You might be worried about what is written here. This could be with good cause, but don't over-react. The first thing to do is make contact with a biological dentist, as they call themselves. These are advanced dentists who appreciate Price's work and freely use homeopathic remedies, nutrition and other natural accompaniments to dental hygiene. They also willingly interact with EAV practitioners, preferring the body's own signals for guidance.

Read more and become informed about the issues. Everyone should take responsibility for their own health care and this applies equally to dentistry. To leave decisions solely to your dentist, if he or she is of conventional thought mode, is to be subject to yesterday's science and it may do you harm in the long run, as we have seen with the mercury story (there remain dentists who *still* insist there is no problem with mercury amalgams).

Eat a proper diet which avoids sugars that cause dental decay and feed micro-organisms. Increase your intake of alkalizing foods to counter any chronic acidosis problem, as discussed in Chapter 11.

Use co-enzyme Q10 supplements (ubiquinone). This has been shown to have unequivocal benefit for periodontal (gum) disease. More teeth are lost due to gum disease than decay (cavities).

Large doses of vitamin C seem to be very helpful for periodontal disease and toxicity of all kinds. Take large amounts before, during and after any dental programme – at least 10 g (2½ teaspoonsful) daily.

CHAPTER 13

THE MOVING
HAND WRITES

The moving hand writes and, having written ... soon goes out of date! Advances in medical bio-electronics are happening very quickly.

One experiment published since this book was commissioned was remarkably successful at showing the necessary existence of an energetic aura which protects the body's own lymphocytes (white blood cells) and is therefore vital for immunity and survival.

Roger Coghill of Pontypool in the UK, co-operating with researcher Tamara Golonja, took human white blood cells and placed them in nutrient fluid in a mu-metal sealed container (mu-metal is a strong barrier to radiations). This container was then strapped to the donor's body (that is, the person from whom the white blood cells had been taken) for 24 hours, with a wire collecting body energy radiations and leading these into the container. After a day had elapsed, the white blood cells were tested for viability using a standard trypan blue exclusion test. If the dye can penetrate the cell membrane it means the cells have been damaged, and the damaged cells turn blue in varying degrees. Intact cells stay colourless. In this test, 70 per cent of the cells remained viable.

As a control, an identical population of white blood cells was placed in another mu-metal sealed container and also strapped to the donor's body, but this time without the wire. Only 50 per cent of cells remained viable, thus showing that in the first case the body had been producing some vital energetic emanation which was capable of travelling down a wire and bringing support to the white blood cells.[1] One would hope the ghosts of Abrams and Boyd were watching (see Chapter 1).

The experiment was further refined by strapping a container population of white blood cells to a non-donor, again with the wire. As before, only 50 per cent survived. So *whose* energy field it was mattered greatly. Finally, to be sure that any old energy was not helpful to cells in this predicament, various electromagnetic fields were tried but the cells still died at the unprotected rate. Indeed, even if the electric fields were of very low intensity, they could actually prove harmful.

Coghill has entered the mobile phone debate by showing that after eight hours' exposure to mobile phones in standby mode the viability of the lymphocytes is markedly reduced compared with unexposed controls, this time by 16.7 per cent three hours after cessation of exposure, and by 23.3 per cent when measured a day later, *even though the cells were not further exposed*. If the phone-exposed cells were compared with the cells exposed to donor fields, the loss of viability was even more pronounced at 32.1 per cent loss and 52.2 per cent loss (next day).

The implications of this simple but sound study are profound: it uncovers for the first time that the natural regulating energetic fields in the body, originating in the brain and elsewhere, have an important direct beneficial influence on our white blood cells. Mental depression and trauma is known to suppress immune function and thereby increase the likelihood of cancer, but this is the first experimental support for the idea that the brain can influence such cells directly without hormones nor via neural pathways. In surgical operations where a lot of blood is lost, the precious white blood cells of the patient could by this technique be saved and nurtured electromagnetically to assist in the recuperation process. The study also adds to the accumulating evidence that though weak radiations from mobile phones pose a health risk, the risks can be mitigated by use of protective devices.

MORE MORA!

Anthony Scott-Morley, already introduced as a world-class EAV specialist (page 89), has recently expressed dissatisfaction with the Vega system and is uncomfortable about the degree of nonreproducibility in EAV testing in general. He presently has the new MORA system which he considers possibly the best machine of the EDS group. His concern with EAV, which I share, is that many patients return values which are generally quite elevated, yet feel perfectly well. On the Voll model, they ought to be suffering from latent or hidden inflammatory disease. Either it exists and we are missing it, or the patients are not really ill. In which case, what do the raised levels mean? Even more disconcertingly, there are patients on whom we obtain normal reads, yet the patient is subsequently discovered to have serious pathology, even cancer.

Scott-Morley addressed himself in some detail to these apparently paradoxical findings. Fortunately, here is a practitioner of several decades' standing, well aware of the capability of these Virtual Medicine systems. He knew there had to be an explanation for the occasional exception, rather than dumping the whole theory. He began to search.

One of his first discoveries was that the temporo-mandibular joint (TMJ), the articulation of the mandible with the skull just in front of the ear, is a critical element in some cases. This arose from observing that the wisdom teeth, which lie across the heart meridian, are an occasional cause of high heart readings among young people whose wisdom teeth have not erupted. The tooth disturbs the energy flow along the heart meridian and gives a false picture. Scott-Morley reasoned that the TMJ was close by and might do the same thing. Subsequent testing confirmed that TMJ displacement can give falsely high readings on any or all of the meridians.

However, there were still unsatisfactory anomalies. Scott-Morley went on investigating, certain there must be answers. He next began to concentrate on the spin phenomenon (see Chapter 3), agreeing very much with what I have described on page 42. Healthy tissues and fluids should be right-spin and toxic or waste substances, such as urine and faeces, should be left-spin. When the 'wrong spin' was corrected, then reading values tended to return to normal. Coincidentally, he made the empirical observation that incorrect polarity often rendered the patient highly susceptible to the influence of electromagnetic fields. He has speculated that the phenomenon we call geopathic stress is actually secondary to incorrect spin; the patient would not be harmfully influenced by such fields if it were not for a pre-existing incorrect spin polarity. Scott-Morley is worth quoting further in this context:

It is clear to me that this phenomenon of polarity is deserving of disciplined scientific investigation. I believe that prevention of reversal of blood polarity may prevent cancer; that manufacture of nutritional supplements such as vitamins and other nutrition products may well be enhanced by right polarity. Manufacture of pharmaceuticals with right polarity may help avoid some of the adverse side effects, and that commercial food production would enhance nutritional value by avoiding left polarity.[2]

These are the deductions of a skilful and informed mind which I am happy to repeat here for my readers to consider.

Finally, Scott-Morley has gone on to evolve a newer model of EAV and bioresonance which I find compelling and practical. He has shared it with other European MORA specialists (being a long-time friend of Morell's son-in-law Erich Rasche) and there is now an exciting concurrence that it is a meaningful breakthrough. The concept is one of 'layers' of chronic disease. It evolved from a unique facility of the MORA, which is the ability to amplify endogenous signals and play these back to the body (page 94). Scott-Morley found that there is a series of definite amplification factors which have a critical beneficial effect on the Voll balance scale of 50.

A neutral (non-EAV) point, such as the ball of the thumb, is chosen and will usually read 50. Body signals are then collected via the other hand electrode and pumped into the reference point at an amplification of 100 (the maximum available). The point will unsettle and the reading will rise to, say, 80. The amplification factor is then reduced successively by 5 to 95, 90, 85, 80, etc., repeating the EAV measurement each time. From 10 on down the amplification is reduced one step at a time: 9, 8, 7 ... 1. For reasons that are not clear, it is observed that three of these critical amplifications will bring the reference point reading back

to the optimum balance of 50. To give an example, for one
patient the reading may be 100, 95, 90 ... **45**, 40, 35 ... **25**, 20 ..., **9**,
8 ... 1.

These critical amplifications could be termed levels of chronic
depths, or chronic layers of disturbance. The situation might be
easier to understand from Scott-Morley's own metaphor of a
pond. Ideally the water should be clear all the way down to the
bottom. The first basic set of measurements (the traditional 1:1
amplification) is like examining the surface of the water for
debris. Usually there will be something there but it may not be
clear whether this is harmless debris, like floating leaves, or diagnostic debris floating up from deeper, more contaminated levels.
The measurements taken in reduced amplification stages are like
sampling the pond water at different levels, from the surface right
down to the bottom of the pond. Logically this gives a far more
accurate picture of what the real pond environment is like. The
deeper the 'bad' layer, the more chronic the disease process.

Having established the three layers, the next step is to retest
the control measurement points for all the meridians, using each
of the amplifications in turn (in this example, 45, 25 and 9). What
is observed now is that the initial readings change substantially –
some increase and many go back to normal. Readings found to
remain abnormal in only one or two of the layers are probably
insignificant. But if an abnormal reading persists through all
three amplification layers, *that is where the chief pathology lies.*
This may not be the same indication given by basic 1:1 testing, as
Voll originally developed it. *Any organ which reveals a disturbance in all three levels must be treated as the first priority.*

It is not uncommon to find that the causal organ is not the obvious one in relation to the presenting symptoms. For example, in a
case of asthma the lungs may reveal disturbance on only one
layer but the autonomic nervous system show abnormality at all
three levels. Here one would be fairly certain that the asthma
attacks are triggered when the nerve net which controls breathing
becomes distressed and starts sending faulty messages. In other
words, the lungs are not exactly misbehaving so much as being
given the wrong 'steering' instructions by the brain and nerves.

Once again, establishing the *true* cause of the illness can lead to a more coherent and better treatment strategy than blindly taking steroids or asthma-suppressing drugs.

It should be pointed out that this layered approach disposes of the contentious question of the separator (page 104). It is not used.

THE RUSSIANS

For reasons that are not altogether obvious, the former Soviets are much more open to novel healing studies and the investigation of psychic effects. It may be because a large part of their culture comes to them from the Orient, instead of Europe, where intellectual conventions remain very staid, even reactionary. Or perhaps this great people faced such a cultural upheaval earlier this century that a mere scientific revolution they can comfortably take in their stride!

Much of what has been written about in this text has had direct parallels in Russian science. In Chapter 3 I featured work which made it clear that the Russians readily embrace the Chinese model and have been researching along these lines for decades. I mentioned Gaikin's observation that Kirlian photography flares often appear at acupuncture points (page 49). It is enthralling to report this has gone further with the development of a system called Acuvision, invented by Romen Avagnyan in Moscow. This also uses high frequencies and high-voltage electronics and causes the acupuncture points to become illuminated and visible on the skin. This clearly hearkens back to the emission of Popp's biophotons (page 154). The points are about the size of a pin-head and can only be seen in a darkened room. Apparently there are many more points than appear in classic texts or even Voll's extended system.

To date this device is no more than an interesting medical curiosity. Dr Avagnyan is of the opinion that this phenomenon can be further exploited for diagnostic potential by measuring the intensity of light emitted by the points. It appears that they glow more intensely where there is excess Ch'i energy and are dimmer when the energy is lower than it should be. This is logical and fits in with everything else I have written in these pages.

Work so far has been confined mainly to limb points and also on the ears. It is of note that the Nogier ear acupuncture points stand out particularly well (page 49). There seems to be great potential for some kind of whole-body scanning system.

THE FUTURE IS HERE

A pocket-sized device to defibrillate hearts, treat sports injuries, strokes, angina, back pains and irritable bowel disease (as well as pre-menstrual tension and post-surgical complications) sounds like a large claim. Professor Yacor Revenko stood on a public stage in Sochi in southern Russia at the 5th Annual Convention in July 1998 and stated that he thought there were few diseases which the family of SCENAR medical devices could not treat and often cure. This new system is a revolutionary approach which again combines the technology of orthodox Western medical practise with ancient knowledge of the East.

Background

In 1986 the offspring of a secret military Soviet project finally emerged into the public domain after nearly 20 years of development behind closed doors. One of the results of work created by a leading Russian Radio-Engineering Institute was a device which is beginning to alter dramatically the way healthcare is delivered in Russia. SCENAR is an Acronym for self controlled energo-neuro-adaptive regulation.

The aim is to stimulate the body's own endogenous energies to effect the cure, using as a mediator the brain's own internal pharmacy of neuropeptides. This allows the body its own choice of healing ingredients. Through biofeedback a dialogue is formed between the tissues and the instrument, each new signal evolves as a new output. No two consecutive signals from the device are the same. This allows the treatment to be truly dynamic, adjusting for changes in state of the body through time and in different physiological conditions.

The SCENAR devices arose from a study of an Eastern therapy known as 'zonal contact massage'. The intention had been to develop some way of altering the pressure of the massage, according to skin response (readers will recall that in chapter 3 I described how the dielectric potential of collagen tissue is stimulated by pressure). Equipment was developed to tap magnetic effects from the skin and use these to modulate changes in pressure of the massage. A team of scientists, including 5 research doctors, was involved in the original studies, based in Sochi and Krasnodar. The establishment of a biofeedback mechanism led to the creation of a device whose output would depend on skin energetic response. The term SCENAR was born. It is yet another brilliant marriage of Western electronic technology and Eastern energetic healing skills.

Background

When the Soviet Union decided to send cosmonauts into orbit for prolonged periods, it was clear that they needed to have a means of treating any illnesses that could befall them. Unlike the American system, there were no convenient re-usable shuttles to bring an ailing cosmonaut back to Earth, should the need have arisen. The possibility of incapacitating disease was a major worry.

The pharmaceutical approach was not tenable, bearing in mind the rigorous weight and space limitations and the fact that dug-oriented medicine is based on the principle of one substance for each (potential) condition. Even a very modest medicine range would be weighty. Also, in an environment where recycling of water is such an essential feature, any drug entering the water circulation system would remain, passing through the cosmonaut many times.

This was at a time when the Russian space programme was being watched by the rest of the world and maintaining national prestige was of paramount concern to the Soviet government. It was essential to come up with something radically new. A large team of doctors and engineers was assembled and they were assigned the task of developing the necessary new technology. It had to be light, easy to use and, of course, really effective.

Bioresonance technology was the only extant medical paradigm capable of delivering these stringent requirements. By expanding on the theoretical work of Anohin, particularly in connection with the reticular formation pathways in the brain, the team developed elegant new physiological models, which led to the current range of electronic interactive devices. Two members of the team were subsequently awarded the Order of Lenin (in their terms, equivalent to a Nobel Prize).

Ironically, no SCENAR device has been used in space to date. There were delays caused by the authorities insisting on a waterproofing process. Before this matter was resolved, funds were suddenly stopped at the time of *perestroika*; the so-called space race was called off and the team disbanded. The US began working on combined space projects with the Russians and they introduced the capability of evacuating sick cosmonauts on the shuttle, which meant there was no further need of on-board therapy.

However, four of the original team felt they had designed a very worthwhile system, capable of changing the face of medicine, and decided to take it onto the open market.

The promise of a small hand-held device that seems capable of curing most illness, such as was portrayed in the cult 1970s TV series 'Star Trek', has become a reality.

Operation
The device resembles a TV remote control and is powered by an ordinary 9v. battery. It is placed on the skin of the chest, head, abdomen or any diseased part, where it collects electromagnetic signals. These are then modulated according to the device's programme and played back to the tissues. Essentially, SCENAR is using the patient's own endogenous signals on a cybernetic feedback basis, scanning and re-transmitting many times a second. As described to me, the device 'evolves' a new signal pattern for the disordered tissues, the machine literally entering into an information dialogue with the body. New frequencies and energy patterns are established, which in turn become fresh input signals, to be further modified, and so on. This *output-equals-new-input* is much the way that fractals are generated and thus, biologically-speaking, we seem to be on good ground here. On the premise that disease signals are generally fixed and unnatural,

anything which breaks up the existing order has the capability of disease-busting.

Casebook: Male, 69 years:
This patient was a gardener with suppurating osteomyelitis of the foot which could not be controlled. He was scheduled for an amputation of the lower leg in four days time, largely because of the intractable pain. At the last moment a British SCENAR practitioner was called into attempt a treatment. The device was used bi-laterally for around 30 minutes on the first day.

Next day, the leg was pain-free for the first time in eight months. Later that day another 30-minute treatment was given. By next morning the recovery was so dramatic the amputation was called off. A third treatment was given and seven days after the first SCENAR this man was back at work, digging in the garden. His leg has completely recovered.

Clinical Aspects
The device is very safe; the impulse times are very short. No pain is felt but the patient is usually aware of a tingling sensation while it works. The practitioner seeks for what the Russians term *asymmetry*, meaning something different about the tissue characteristics in the vicinity.

There are five main criteria:

- colour difference (reddening or pallor)
- sensation (numbness or hyper-aesthesia)
- 'stickiness' in which the machine drags with a magnet like quality as it is drawn over certain tracts of the skin
- sound changes (the machine begins to chatter electronically when it hits the right zone)
- Numerical display readings alter

Even though it may not coincide with the obvious area of symptoms or pathology, the important point is to *treat the asymmetry*.

For reasons we do not fully understand, when this is eliminated, recovery will rapidly follow.

Summary

A summary of findings in different clinical groups on 50,000 cases from 3,000 SCENAR users doctors and other practitioners includes cumulative percentages in which ëeffectivenessí is defined as a cure in 66% of cases and some improvement in 33% of cases:

Circulatory	82%
Respiratory	84%
Gastrointestinal	93%
Genito-urinary	89%
Gynae and Obstetrics	78%
Musculoskeletal	79%
Ear and Mastoid	82%
Eye and adnexae	93%
Mouth/jaw/saliva glands	91%

This list is far from exhaustive and I have been able to establish that there are many other areas in which SCENAR is highly effective. For example, there is a current 98% cure rate achievement for benign postatic hypertrophy and in the case of acute mastitis the device is 100% effective to date. Nothing I know of can come close to its figures against frigidity, impotence and infertility (60th percentile).

There are remarkably few contra-indications, notably heart pacemakers and, after 20 years, a complete absence of negative side-effects. SCENAR technology can be used as a valuable addition to other therapies or could be a stand-alone treatment. There extra-ordinary feature is that the same small device can be used to treat the heart of one patient, the knee of the next, the breasts and adnexa of the next - all relying on one small battery as an energy source!

MAGNETIC RESONANCE ON A CREDIT CARD

One of the platforms of this book has been that strange-sounding alternative medicine ideas are often based on sound physics and that conventional science and medicine must endure a process of catching up with the van. So it is with some satisfaction that I report the emergence of a bioresonance diagnostic system developed at the University of Bangor in Wales.[3] This is decades behind Voll and Morell but most welcome, since many authorities tend to assume that a pronouncement from a university has special credence. More to the point, institutions of this type often have vast budgets to spend on investigating something which has tickled the academic fancy; vast, that is, in relation to the paltry sums we have available in the alternative arena for research.

The gimmick is that this device is little bigger than the size of a credit card. Yet by bouncing signals off the body's molecular structure and interpreting the return oscillations, it is able to detect the unique energy 'signatures' of bacteria, antibodies, viruses, hormones and other biological molecules. What makes the signatures identifiable is specific changes in the conductivity of the cell surface. When cells are altered by infection and other disease processes, the cell surface membrane undergoes change in conductivity. By calibrating this effect against known diseases, it is possible to build up a library of signals, just as with the Oscilloclast register or an EDS system database.

As Dr. Julian Burt, research fellow at the university Institute for Molecular and Biomolecular Electronics explains: 'Any particle you put into the electromagnetic field will move. What our technolgy does is to pic up the differences in characteristic molecular substances by measuring how fast and in what direction they race along the electrode arrays'.[3]

With the introduction of this system, I make the point that once we have the right technology it will be possible to dispose of the awkward TCM (acupuncture) element of Voll's system. The key to this is that an energy field, characterized by the information of a pathological process, is like any other field and attenuates to infinity. Although there would be practical difficulties, provided the detectors are sensitive enough you could theoretically do the diagnosis in the next room, never mind any need to touch the body at acupuncture points.

Indeed, I foresee the time when medical diagnosis is simply a matter of the patient walking through a detector loop or gate and the disease process and relevant organ will flash up on a screen, virtually instantaneously. It is not only quite realistic but *very very* close, certainly within the lifetime of the early editions of this book and no more than a decade hence. It would be the final fulfilment of the far-sighted visions of Abrams, Lakhovsky and Crile.

CHAPTER 14

ELECTRONIC KUNDALINI

A view of the new medical paradigm I have called Virtual Medicine would be incomplete without looking at the deeper philosophical implications of what this new domain of knowledge is teaching us. Few doctors to date are even fully aware of the progress that has been made in this field, much less espouse the system of healing it engenders. But nevertheless, there is a clear situation where advances in healing science and technology have led us to a new appreciation of the very meaning of life. Life is no longer merely the flesh. We 'live' outside the skin! To me these new horizons are significant, since it is largely a doctor's role to be expert in these matters and to be able to inform the public about the issues.

I have always felt that the real meaning of healing and 'doctoring' is to be able to see a patient in the wider context as a life form in a big brawling universe and to seek to bring healing at this level. Merely removing or suppressing symptoms is really to miss most of the problem, which is that the patient is out of balance and is experiencing a degree of separation from his or her true place in the cosmos. In this view, disease is just the result of this lack of integration. The traditional shamanic healer knows far more about our true nature and our place in the scheme of things than a scientifically-trained Western 'medicine man'. They understand healing at what I decm to be a far deeper level of awareness than science. The Hollywood cliché portrayal of the witch-doctor as an ignorant savage who is marginalized by a hero who steps in with a life-saving penicillin shot has always seemed to me to be completely backwards. *The fact is that more people on earth get well more of the time by using the safe and traditional healing approach than get well by means of drugs.* The trouble is that doctors see too many such movies and start to believe their own propaganda.

There is much to be ashamed of in the way modern medicine is conducted. I have been involved in many shamanic experiments and can assure the reader that a dramatic 'soul-retrieval' as it is called has often been effective in a cure, where conventional medicine was simply unable to help. Just one of those things, you may suppose. But what nobody needs is the profession which failed to help, scoffing and deriding the one which did! There's no humanity or love in these shows of pique and they do not serve the cause of genuine enquiry.

This book is offered as a small light in the new dawn of which it is but a tiny part. It was also written in the hope that, by sticking fairly close to the scientific model, it will partly persuade those who think otherwise that there are many strange and vital manifestations of life which are not merely illusions. In fact, using the equipment I have described in the previous chapters, one cannot fail to be impressed by the obviousness of mysterious forces that interplay with our lives and give it far more meaning than just the foraging and procreation of a carbon dioxide engine.

I have found these devices to be not merely diagnostic tools but also in a sense learning systems. If only medical students were shown some of the properties of tissues and pathogens that are seen clearly when practising Virtual Medicine it would give them a totally different orientation in their chosen profession. They would gain respect for the divine, the supernormal and the simply awesome characteristics of Nature and life. To see how the human energies kick over when a pathogen is merely brought close to the body is, I always feel, to teach us something about ourselves and our nature, not just the mechanism of disease.

The well-trained doctor of the future may begin to talk a little bit like the shamans or magicians of old, where the central role of manifest reality and the conscious interaction with it is the sole and total basis of life-renewal and healing forces. I don't think that means we will never use antibiotics, anaesthetics, lasers or the other paraphernalia of modern high-tech medicine. But I hope that, through time, the adoption of the techniques and (even more importantly) the principles outlined in this book will become the mainstay of medical practice. I fervently believe that technological medicine now finds itself at a watershed. It is a time of a collective paradigm shift, when professional and scientific attitudes move from one set of truths to another.

STICKING WITH SCIENCE

It has been the purpose of this text to concentrate on objective scientifically-provable facts, albeit novel ones. This is for a very good reason; while it is necessary to demystify these life-phenomena, we must avoid accusing science of being somehow 'wicked'. We should not generalize that everything that matters and is nourishing in healing is somehow superior, other-worldly (even 'divine') and forever beyond our ken. The commonly used mystical and fairy-story rhetoric is proving a serious barrier to wider acceptance of this knowledge by the scientific and medical community.

As Dr Julian Kenyon, co-founder of The Centre for the Study of Complementary Medicine in Southampton, UK, has stated: 'The idea of applying scientific measurement to energetic parameters has not been greeted with enthusiasm by the often doctrinaire proponents of skills such as traditional Chinese medicine and classical homeopathy in particular. Many of these disciplines are surrounded by some degree of mystique, a proportion of which does not stand up to critical examination.'[1]

It might be assumed that I am taking a position here which does not believe in the divine manifestation of life or that there is nothing beyond physics, nothing we can call the soul or spirit, no God or no ineffable quality of it all. Not so. Indeed, the opposite. I care passionately about the life immortal and the nature of what may be termed 'transcendental'. I have spent years researching past-life phenomena as part of healing and have mounted a project I call *Tunnels of Time* here in Spain.

KEY QUESTION

Where does the boundary of theoretical physics end and the transcendental begin? Is it a sharp boundary or is there a gradual blurring from ordinary reality to mystical consciousness? One would also be justified in wondering if the threshold actually moves and, if so, under what circumstances? Or is it perhaps always fixed and a matter of divine construct? These are meaty questions but it seems to me that those of us at the cutting edge should be asking them. The time is right for that 'quantum shift' into the Age of Aquarian consciousness, which may be our gift to the coming generations, as much as the Renaissance was to those from the 14th century onwards. I do not know the answer to any of the boundary questions, but just to ask them and appreciate their significance is intellectually stimulating.

Is our world the property of our consciousness, or the other way round?

This blurring of the boundary between the properties of mind and theoretical physics was the theme of a general public wake-up in the late 1970s, occasioned by popular texts such as *The Dancing Wu-Li Masters* by Gary Zukov and *The Tao of Physics* by Fritjof Capra. Both authors brought together the existing knowledge of the mysterious world of quantum physics and showed how closely our present understanding of the supposedly objective and 'real' world paralleled the postulated creation of existence described long ago in the Sanskrit Vedas and the Pali canon. One was indeed impressed by the striking convergence of two (apparently) alien intellectual streams.

It was, as I said earlier in the present text, a matter of science catching up with esoteric wisdom, rather than the other way round. I think Einstein's metaphor is even more apposite:

... creating a new theory is not like destroying an old barn and erecting a skyscraper in its place. It is rather like climbing a mountain, gaining new and wider views, discovering unexpected connections between our starting point and its rich environment. But *the point from which we started out still exists* and can still be seen, although it appears smaller and forms a tiny part of our broad view gained by the mastery of the obstacles on our adventurous way up.[2]

THOUGHT MACHINES

One of science's fashions is to chase the grail of computers which can think like humans. The so-called Turing Test, named after British mathematician Alan Turing, is supposed to define the moment at which a machine can actually 'think' or at least appear to think by fooling the observers.

Another more important search is under way, a kind of electronic holism and, so far, Big Business is leaving it to those who care. We may soon have machines which embody *real* human thought, in other words machines which are a composite of physical matter and human mind. The fact is, the horizon between consciousness and physical reality is fast becoming so blurred I predict that within the first dozen years of the next millennium we will have computers which can interact directly with thought.

It will depend on two directions of progress: expanding our consciousness, making it more intensely coherent, and the development of small-scale electronics which are capable of sensing changes in our thought processes. Both pre-requisites are well advanced.

Boffins and engineers have attempted to expand the physical limitations of computing, trying to devise new ways to get more and more computing power using fewer and fewer physical resources. Electronics hardware systems have shrunk by half approximately every 18 months in the past 20 years. If this trend continues, soon individual electronic logic gates (the decision points that once upon a time were clumsy transistors) will be down to the size of atoms, and currents will be measured in terms of the number of electrons which move. There is no theoretical reason this cannot come about; it is merely a question of the present technical difficulties.[3]

The problem is that, when computer systems are so small, reliability reaches its practical limit. Nano-electronics operations become subject to disruption by 'noise' or extraneous interference. There are surprising new sources of such noise, including mysterious alpha-particle 'pollution' from unknown sources, which continue to challenge the limitations of practical physics.

It seems likely the human thought processes can also become 'noise' and disrupt computations. We have already seen from Chapter 2 that the brain and mind processes can give off magnetic fields detectable by SQUIDS. It is only a matter of time before this effect is harnessed and deliberate connection of thought energy processes to a computer becomes a reliable reality.

To solve problems in this complex area of nano-electronics, scientists have begun to study the relationship between information and other laws of physics. This understanding is incomplete but lies within the tantalizing domain of probabilistic quantum theory. We talk a lot about information fields, which are now much the fashion. Yet most people forget that implicit in the term 'information' is the notion of consciousness. Advanced physicists are putting the concept of living and awareness back into the structure of the cosmos.

And of course information or consciousness brings us back to the other requirement for interactive machines, which is coherent field broadcasting by the mind with sufficient power.

KUNDALINI AWAKENING

How can we seek to strengthen our consciousness and what criteria evince any improvement? Historically, our Western culture has viewed consciousness in the same order of reference as intelligence. The supposition is that more mental power means more storage and retrieval from contents of a warehouse or database somewhere within the mind. It is a computer-oriented view and is fine as far as it goes. *But it has nothing whatever to do with consciousness.* The very same comparison with computers proves the point: to have a massive memory and algorithmic capability does not imply any awareness of the process going on in one's silicon guts.

Gradually we are being forced to look at a more holistic paradigm, for the psyche and for reality. The new model of consciousness is one of information or constructive input into experience. I could not presume to define consciousness, but I think I am not exactly out on a limb in saying that it clearly implies some participative interaction with reality. It is about the *actual* experience and not the logging or recording of experience, as in the cyber domain. In other words it centres around perception and not memory.

Thus anything which increases perception ability is valid material with which to expand consciousness.

Traditional Eastern meditative practices have always utilized a rather passive and dissociative aim in relation to developing finer consciousness. The assumption is that by quieting the 'chatter' within the mind, the greater consciousness will emerge, rather like a timid fawn creeping out of the forest where it has hidden. Isolation tank research has tended to support this view, where 'less' means 'more'. Subjects describe inspired new levels of perception and feeling when once the noise within falls silent. Biofeedback techniques also seem to work better when the subject gives up trying and just relaxes in expectation.

There are two main problems with this traditional passive approach: it takes too long and it does not focus with coherence sufficient to be likely to waken up an electronics system. Some newer approach is required. Interesting new possibilities are emerging all the time. I already referred in Chapter 9 (Caduceus) to the induction of *samadhi* using gem-stressed light and suitable frequencies. The Monroe Institute has taken this theme much further and can create out-of-the-body experiences, using music, rhythms and flashing lights. New dynamics are being evolved by research groups all over the world.

It isn't too fanciful to liken this to an awakening of an electronic kundalini, the power within the cosmos inherent in our Being.

BOHM'S BRAVE NEW WORLD

On a final serious note, while writing of the increasingly hazy demarcation between mind perception and so-called objective reality, it is essential to mention David Bohm's holographic universe concept. It is only a metaphor but it is an exciting one and it could well contain the essential truth needed to integrate organic wholeness, what is Divine and the epistemology of perception. The proper union of these three elements of philosophy has eluded scientists and thinkers since the dawn of thinking. How does Bohm's hypothesis help?

First, let me explain an important point about holograms. Everyone knows that you can see them in three dimensions; it is a means of visualizing an object as a volume solid and is used in museums to preserve valuable specimens intact while allowing them to be appreciated by visitors. What is less well known, but is actually a far more important property of holograms, is that each part contains the whole. If you take a pair of scissors and cut a hologram in two, both halves contain the full picture. If you cut it in half again, each new fragment still contains the whole picture. This can go on indefinitely; no matter how small the piece, it still contains the whole image, though obviously it becomes fainter and fainter as the representational elements become smaller and smaller.

Bohm's novel insight was to suppose that physical reality may be constructed in some similar fashion. In other words, the universe itself acts as a hologram. Bohm called the picture we see *the explicate order* (from explicit), and the hidden total inner picture *the implicate order* (from implicit or hidden).[4] What does this actually mean? Well, if Bohm's idea is correct, it means that all parts of existence are contained in each tiny fragment. The desk on which my word processor stands has all the elements of creation and reality, from the dawn of time to the end of the universe; every atom, every galaxy. If I unscrew one of the drawer handles and inspect it, even *that* could contain the totality of everything! This is an appalling thought, but at the same time a thrilling one.

Certain threads from the Virtual Medicine paradigm now begin to converge. For example, we saw that Sheldrake's morphogenic fields are something super-ordinary; something above the range of energy and matter, that acted as a kind of blueprint. Could these fields be part of the implicate order? If so, does it not mean that DNA, that wonder chemical substance that contains the codes for living organisms, could be the life-bridge between the implicate and explicate orders? Remember Roger Coghill's suggestion that the DNA molecule works as a transmitter aerial on page 21. But what does it transmit? Radio waves? Or some bolder cosmic message of order and creation?

The mind itself, of course, will form part of that bridge to reality. Information, as I have said before, *implies* consciousness and awareness. You can't have one without the other. This is a potential paradox solved by reference to the Eastern sages and the British Empiricist philosophers: what we are is a product of what we perceive and vice versa. There is no difference between the perceiver and the perceived.

Nobody knows if Bohm's hypothesis is the final answer, but in terms of consistency it is a hard theory to beat, because almost all mysteries of the world we experience become understandable in simple terms of explicit versus implicit order. Take telepathy or past lives as examples. If all of existence is wrapped up in every little fragment of reality, that would also include the matter inside our brains. Any piece of the brain has the whole of the rest of reality wrapped up in it somewhere (I am purposely side-stepping the fact that *mind* is unlikely to be exactly congruent with *brain*). We can potentially know everything, all in an instant. Now that's what ancient sages have been saying, so the idea is not so alien. What is new is a means to understand how this could be true. Bohm's brave new universe is very satisfying in many respects.

The corollary is that, if we know everything, then we have to selectively un-know things, otherwise our consciousness would just go into overdrive and ... well, who knows what? We can speculate.

THE LAST WORD

Let's end on a lighter note by taking Virtual Medicine to the extreme outer fringe. It has been postulated that man may one day abandon his flesh body and become so integrated with computers that our personality resides entirely within the software of the cyber domain. This would be *virtual living*, rather than the virtual reality being debated today; consciousness would be in the computer world looking out into what we assume to be reality, instead of the other way round.

Celebrated writer Arthur C. Clarke first put forward this idea in a 1956 book *The City and the Stars*, though how the fictional civilization managed this trick he does not reveal in the story. But writer Bob Ettinger takes it very seriously and his book *Man Into Superman* is definitely non-fiction.[5] He foresees the day when it will be possible to transfer our human personalities to a software package which thinks, feels and communicates. We would then dispense with the inconvenient restrictions of the body and its incessant demands for foraging and procreation. Should such a scenario ever come to pass, we would of course be 'immortal', though there would need to be back-up copies for safety. These back-up personalities would have to be updated regularly, otherwise they would become invalid because they were missing too many experiences. Ed Regis, author of *Great Mambo Chicken and the Transhuman Condition* (which for both our sakes I had better state is subtitled *Science Slightly Over the Edge*) calls this state *post-biological man*.[6] You might worry that, even if you felt you were now inside a computer – that you were *really* there – you would no longer be able to experience anything real. Any input sensations would be mere simulation. Well, according to David Hume, greatest of the British Empiricists referred to above, that's all you ever get in life anyway! All of living is only a mind simulation of whatever is 'out there' (if anything).

It may come as a shock to readers to realize that these ideas are being seriously debated. Do not be tempted to scoff at this possibility of cyber-life. It may be closer than you think. 'What Nature can do,' Arthur C. Clarke wrote, 'Man can also do in his own way.' As Frederik Pohl, also a sci-fi writer, stated in a 1964 *Playboy* article entitled 'Intimations of Immortality': 'The essential "you" isn't your body. It is what we call your personality, your memory, your mind. This essential "you" could be preserved inside a computer, a collection of magnetic impulses in an IBM computer.'[7]

What then would be the state of Virtual Medicine?

Presumably physicians like me would have to be computer geeks and know how to handle floppy discs, save, copy, back-up, restore and edit files. Illness might then be a question of corrupted memory or glitches and we would have to put this right. A major operation would be to shut down the computer system and re-instal you from a back-up. By then evolution would be reduced to thinking up newer and better software packages to broadcast ourselves from.

This prospect makes Aldous Huxley's *Brave New World* seem like a vicarage tea party. But if in the far distant future it came about, and there just happened to be a mouldering centuries-old copy of this book found on a forgotten shelf somewhere, no-one will be able to turn to the last page and read those foolish words: IT COULD NEVER HAPPEN!

RESOURCES

PREFACE
1 F. Capra, *The Tao of Physics*.

CHAPTER 1
1 A. Linde, 'The Self-Reproducing Inflationary Universe', *Scientific American* vol 9, no. 1, 1998.
2 M. White, *Isaac Newton, The Last Sorcerer* (Fourth Estate, 1997).
3 R. Sheldrake, *The Rebirth of Nature* (Rider, 1990).
4 J. C. Eccles, *Evolution of the Brain: Creation of the Self* (Routledge, 1989).
5 R. D. Pearson, *Intelligence Behind the Universe* (The Headquarters Publishing Co. Ltd., 1990).
6 R. Gerber, *Vibrational Medicine* (Santa Fe, NM: Bear, 1988).
7 A. Abrams, *New Concepts in Diagnosis and Treatment* (San Francisco: Philopolis Press, 1916).
8 K. Mumby, 'Science or Flat Earthers?', *British Medical Journal* 307 (23rd October 1993): 1055–6.
9 H. Gaier (ed), *Thorsons Encyclopaedic Dictionary of Homeopathy* (Thorsons, 1991).
10 R. O. Becker, *Cross Currents: The Perils of Electropollution, The Promise of Electromedicine* (NY: Tarcher/Putnam, 1990): 239.
11 J. R. Thomas, J. Schrot and A. Liboff, 'Production of passive behaviour in mice by means of lithium cyclotron resonance', *Biomagnetics* 7 (1986): 349.

CHAPTER 2
1 H. Schiegl, *Healing Magnetism* (Century, 1987): 13.
2 H. S. Burr, *Blueprint for Immortality* (Saffron Walden: C W Daniel and Co, 1972).
3 Ibid.
4 G. Lakhovsky, *The Secret of Life* (True Health Publishing Co, 1951 [English translation copyright 1970 by Mark Clement]): 3.

5 Ibid.
6 K. Mumby, *The Complete Guide to Allergy and Environmental Illness* (Thorsons, 1993).
7 A. Nodon, 'Les nouvelles radiations ultra-pénétrantes et à cellule vivante', *Revue Scientifique* 22nd October 1927: 609.
8 Lakhovsky, op cit. 111.
9 R. O. Becker, *The Body Electric* (Morrow, New York 1985).
10 J. L. Oschman, 'What Is Healing Energy? Part 2: Measuring the Fields of Life', *Journal of Bodywork and Movement Therapies* January 1997: 117–22.
11 R. Sheldrake, *New Science of Life* (Rider, 1990).

CHAPTER 3

1 Chang Tsai, quoted in Fung Yu-lan, *A Short History of Chinese Philosophy* (NY: Macmillan, 1958): 279.
2 Sir T. Lewis, 'The Nocifensor System of Nerves and its Reactions', *British Medical Journal* 27th February 1937: 431.
3 P. de Vernejoul *et al.*, 'Etude Des Méridiens D'Acupuncture par les Traceurs Radioactifs', *Bull. Acad. Natle. Med.* vol. 169 (22nd October, 1985): 1071—5.
4 R. O. Becker, *Cross Currents: The Perils of Electropollution, The Promise of Electromedicine* (NY: Tarcher/Putnam, 1990): 90.
5 H. Motoyama, *Theories of the Chakras* (IL: Theosophical Publishing House, 1981).
6 Hunt Dr. V, Massey W, Weinberg R, Bruyere R, and Hahn P., *'Project Report, A Study of Structural Integration from Neuromuscular, Energy Field and Emotional Approches.'* U.C.L.A., 1977.
7 D. J. Matzke, 'Prediction: Future Electronics Will Be Disrupted due to Consciousness', paper at *Towards a Science of Consciousness* conference, Tucson II, University of Arizona, 1996.
8 J. R. Wosley, *Everyone's Guide to Acupuncture* (Cassell, 1973): 43.
9 Ibid: 44.
10 M. Wexu, *The Ear, Gateway to Balancing the Body: A Modern Guide to Acupuncture* (NY: ASI Publishers, 1975).
11 K. Mumby, *The Allergy Handbook* (Thorsons, 1989).

CHAPTER 4

1 Stortebecker P. *Dental Caries as a Cause of Nervous Disorders*, Bio-Probe Inc, Orlando, USA, 1986. P. 39.
2 R. Voll, 'The Phenomenon of Medicine Testing in Electroacupuncture According to Voll', *Am Acupunct* 8, 1980: 97–104.

REFERENCE

3 K.-G. Chen, 'Applying Quantum Interference to EDST Medicine Testing', *IEEE Engineering in Medicine and Biology* (four-part series) May/June 1996: 64–6.
4 J Benveniste, 'The Memory of Molecules', *The Independent* Friday Review, 19th March 1999.
5 J. J. Tsuei, C. W. Lehman, F. Lam Jr, D. Zhu, 'A Food Allergy Study Utilizing the EAV Acupuncture Technique', *Am J Acupunct* 12, 1984: 105–16.
6 P. Chou, J. J. Tsuei, C. H. Chen, 'Clinical Application of Bioenergy in the Cardiovascular System', report to the ROC National Research Institute of Chinese Medicine, 1985: NRICM-84–103.
7 Dr Julian Kenyon, personal communication June 1998, in the form of a draft chapter of a forthcoming book.

CHAPTER 5

1 R. Van Wijk and F. A. C. Wilegart, 'Homeopathic Remedies and Pressure-induced Changes in Galvanic Resistance of the Skin', Dept of Molecular Biology, State University of Utrecht, Research Unit for Complementary Medicine, Padualaan 8, 3584 CH Utrecht, 1989.
2 R. Van Wijk, 'Homeopathic Medicines in Closed Phials Tested by Changes in the Conductivity of the Skin: A Critical Evaluation. Blind Testing and Partial Elucidation of the Mechanisms', Dept of Molecular Biology, State University of Utrecht, Research Unit for Complementary Medicine, Padualaan 8, 3584 CH Utrecht, 1992.
3 J. Kenyon, *21st Century Medicine* (Thorsons, 1986).
4 D. J. Matzke, 'Prediction: Future Electronics Will Be Disrupted due to Consciousness', paper at *Towards a Science of Consciousness* conference, Tucson II, University of Arizona, 1996.
5 Lawden DF, Separability of Psycho-physical Systems, Psycho-Energetics. The Journal of Psycho-physical Systems, vol 4, no 1, 1-10 (1981).

CHAPTER 6

1 E. Rasche, *Elektronische Homeopathie* (Friesenheim: Medtronik Trading GmbH, 1998).
2 H. Gaier (ed), *Thorsons Encyclopaedic Dictionary of Homeopathy* (Thorsons, 1991): 57
3 Quoted in H. Brügemann (ed), *Bioresonance and Multiresonance Therapy* (vol 1; Haug: Brussels, 1990 [English edn, 1993]).
4 Rasche, op cit
5 Brügemann, op cit

CHAPTER 7

1 E. Hamlyn, *The Healing Art of Homeopathy* (The Organon of Samuel Hahnemann, Beaconsfield Publishers, 1979).
2 L. Watson, *Supernature* (Hodder and Stoughton, 1973).
3 Davenas E, Benveniste J et al. 'Human basophil degranulation triggered by very dilute antiserum against IgE, *Nature 333* (1988):816; 1988..
4 H.-H. Reckeweg, *Homotoxicology – illness and healing through anti-homotoxic therapy* (Albuquerque, NM: Menaco Publishing Co, 1980).
5 A. Pischinger, *Matrix and Matrix Regulation, Basis for a Holistic Theory in Medicine* (Brussels: Haug International, 1986).
6 H. Gaier (ed), *Thorsons Encyclopaedic Dictionary of Homeopathy* (Thorsons, 1991): 66.
7 S. Bawin and W. R. Adey, 'First report of ELF fields producing calcium efflux from nerve cells', *Proceedings of the National Academy of Sciences* 73 (1976): 1999.
8 van Wijk R, et al, A Molecular Basis for Understanding the Benefits from Subharmful Doses of Toxicatns, *Environmental Management and Health*, Vol 5 No. 1, 1994, pp 13–25..
9 Personal communication from George Burns, Manchester homeopath.
10 Gaier, op cit: 345.
11 K Mumby, *The Allergy Handbook* (Thorsons, 1989).
12 E Bach and F J Wheeler, *The Bach Flower Remedies* (New Canaan, CT: Keats, 1977).
13 E. Rasche, *Elektronische Homeopathie* (Friesenheim: Medtronik Trading GmbH, 1998).
14 J Benveniste, 'The Memory of Molecules', *The Independent* Friday Review, 19th March 1999.

CHAPTER 8

1 K. Mumby, *The Allergy Handbook* (Thorsons, 1989).
2 J. Diamond and L. W. Cowden, *The Alternative Medicine Definitive Guide to Cancer* (Tiburon, CA: Future Medicine Publishing Inc., 1997): 1027.

CHAPTER 9

1 Szent-Gyorgi, Introduction to a Sub-Moledular Biology, *Academic Press*, New York, 1960.
2 Berezin Martinez, Artificial Light-Sensitive Enzyme Systems as Chemical AMplifiers of Weak Light Signals, *Photochemistry Photobiology .29*, March 1979, pp637-650.

3   F. A. Popp, 'New Avenues in Medicine' (two-part radio broadcast in the series *Neues Aus Kultur und Wissenschaft*; Deutschlandfunk Radio, Aug–Sept 1979. Published in H Brügemann (ed), *Bioresonance and Multiresoance Therapy* (vol 1; Haug: Brussels, 1990 [English edn, 1993]).

4   J Liberman Light: Medecine of the Future, Bear and Co, Santa Fe, 1991, p51.

5   Beral V, et al.,'Malignant melanoma and exposure to fluorescent light' Lancet 2 (1982) pp 290-292.

6   B. Bhattacharya, *Gem Therapy* (Calcutta: Firma KLM Private Ltd, 1993).

7   T. Engineer, P. Richards, 'VRIC Imaging the Photon', paper presented at the International Forum of New Science, Denver, Colorado, 1997.

8   T. Engineer, 'Biolumanetics – The Science of Life-Light', *Positive Health* March 1998: 23–7.

CHAPTER 10

1   R. O. Becker, *Cross Currents: The Perils of Electropollution, The Promise of Electromedicine* (NY: Tarcher/Putnam, 1990): 182.

2   K. Mumby, *The Complete Guide to Food Allergy and Environmental Illness* (Thorsons, 1993): 193.

3   Ibid: 69.

4   R. Coghill, *Something in the Air* (Coghill Research Laboratories, Lower Race, Gwent NP4 5UH, Wales, 1997).

5   Dr B. Kohler, 'The Basic Principles of Multiresonance Therapy with Biologically Effective Environmental Signals', in H Brügemann (ed), *Bioresonance and Multiresoance Therapy* (vol 1; Haug: Brussels, 1990 [English edn 1993]).

6   K. Mumby, *The Allergy Handbook* (Thorsons, 1989).

7   Becker, op cit: 302.

8   J. Pawlik, P. Chase, *Newcastle Guide to Healing with Crystals* (North Hollywood, CA: Newcastle Publishing Co, 1988).

9   Mumby, op cit.

CHAPTER 11

1   L. Roujon, *Theory and Practice of the Bio-electric 'Vincent'* (SIBEV, 1975).

2   S. W. Seldin and G. Giebisch, *The Regulation of Acid-Base Balance* (NY: Raven Press, 1989).

3   A. Guyton, *Textbook of Medical Physiology* (Philadelphia: W. B. Saunders, 1991).

4   B. Bandy and A. J. Davison, 'Mitochondrial Mutations May Increase Oxidative Stress: Implications for Carcinogenesis and Ageing?' *Free Radical Biology and Medicine* 8 (1990): 823–39.

5   W. M. Clark, *Oxidation-Reduction Potentials of Organic Systems* (Baltimore: The Williams & Wilkins Company, 1960).

6   P. Wingate, C. Gifford and R. Treays, *Essential Science* (Tulsa, OK: EDC Publishing, 19xx — TO COME).

7   Guyton, op cit.

8   Published circular by Dr Jeffrey Klass, 625 East Main Street, Branford, Connecticut 06405, USA.

CHAPTER 12

1   J. D. Beck, S. Offenbacher, R. Williams, P. Gibbs and R. Garcia, 'Periodontitis: A Risk Factor for Coronary Heart Disease?', *Annals of Periodontology* vol. 3, no. 1, July 1998: 127–41.

2   Stortebecker P. Dental Caries as a Cause of Nervous Disorders, Bio-Probe Inc, Orlando, USA, 1986. P74.

3   Stortebecker P. Dental Caries as a Cause of Nervous Disorders, Bio-Probe Inc, Orlando, USA, 1986. P34.

4   Ibid: p.116.

5   R. Turk, 'Iatrogenic Damage Due to High-speed Drilling', paper presented at the Scientific Session at the dedication of the Princeton Bio Center, New Jersey, 13th June, 1981.

6   H. Raue, 'Resistance to Therapy; Think of Tooth Fillings', *Medical Practice* vol 32, no 72, 6th September 1980: 2303——9.

7   J. E. Bouquot, *In Review of Nico, G V Black's Forgotten Disease*, The Maxillofacial Centre, 583 Tibbs Rd, Morgantown, West Virginia, Third Edition, 1995.

8   G. Meinig, *Root Canal Cover-up* (Ojai, CA: Bion Publishing, 1995).

9   Radio interview of the *Laura Lee Show*, transcript published in the *Townsend Letter for Doctor and Patient* August/September 1996.

CHAPTER 13

1   R. Coghill, T. Golonja, 'Viability of human lymphocytes exposed to endogenous electric fields of the donor'. Results first presented at the Bio-electromagnetics Society meeting, Florida, June 1998.

2   A. Scott-Morley, 'Bioinformation Therapy: Some New Thoughts' (article circulated via e-mail: electrodoc@demon.co.uk

3   'Lab o chip gives instant diagnosis of illness' Sunday Times, 27 September 1998..

CHAPTER 14

1 Dr Julian Kenyon, personal communication in the form of a draft chapter for a book on Bio-Energetic regulatory medicine, October 1998.

2 Quoted in G. Zukov, *The Dancing Wu-Li Masters* (publication information TO COME).

3 D. J. Matzke, 'Prediction: Future Electronics Will Be Disrupted due to Consciousness', paper at *Towards a Science of Consciousness*, Tucson II, University of Arizona, 1996.

4 M. Talbot, *The Holographic Universe* (HarperCollins, 1996).

5 R. C. W. Ettinger, *Man Into Superman* (NY: St Martin's Press, 1972).

6 E. Regis, *Great Mambo Chicken and the Transhuman Condition* (Penguin Science, 1992).

7 Quoted in Regis, op cit.

USEFUL ADDRESSES

Please note: If dialling a US number from outside the US, please add the prefix 00–1. If dialling a UK number from outside the UK, please add the prefix 011–44 and omit the first 0. If dialling a German number from outside Germany, please add the prefix 011–49 and omit the first 0.

American Association of Acupuncture and Bioenergetic Medicine
2512 Manoa Road
Honolulu, HI 96822
USA
Tel: (808) 946-2069
Fax: (808) 946-0378

Field Mouse
Coghill Research Laboratories
Lower Race
Pontypool, Gwent NP4 5UH
Wales
UK
Tel: 01495 767755
Fax: 01495 769882

Mora Machine
MED-Tronik GmbH
Daimlerstrasse 2
D-7632 Friesenheim
Germany

BICOM Machine
Regumed
Lochhamer Schlag 5a
D-82166 Gräfelfing
Tel: 089 854 6102
089 854 6103

Caduceus Machine
Whale Medical
5, Church Hill
Arnside
Cumbria LA5 0DQ
UK
Tel: 01542 762526

Biolumanetics
Thrity Engineer, 3-S
199 Mortlake Road
Kew
Surrey TW9 4EW
UK
Tel/Fax: 0181 878 6693

Biological Terrain Machines
Biological Technologies
International
PO Box 560
Payson, AZ 85547
USA
Tel: (520) 474-4181
Fax: (520) 474-1501

Russian SCENAR
Philip Barker
Tinneys Firs
Redlynch
Wiltshire
UK

Scott-Mumby Clinics
Box 221
Mijas 29650
Malaga
Spain
Tel/Fax: (34) 95 266 1207
In the UK: 0700 078 1744
email: scottmumby@jet.es

Anthony Scott-Morley
103, North Road
Parkstone
Poole
Dorset BH14 0LU
UK
Tel/Fax: 01202 733762
email: electrodoc@aol.com

BEST System and LISTEN System
BioMeridian
216 North Orem Boulevard
Orem, UT 84057
USA
Tel: (888) 224-2337/(801) 226-1117
Fax: (801) 226-1147
email: mail@biomeridian.com

Futureplex
Vega Test Ampoules
Staufen-Pharma GmbH & Co.
Postfach 1143
D-73011 Göppingen
Germany
Tel: 07161-676-0
Fax: 07161-676-298

Vega Machines
Vega Grieshaber KG
Postfach 1142
D-77757 Schiltach
Germany
Tel: 07836-50219
Fax: 07836-50206

Complex Homeopathy Suppliers
Heel Complex Homeopathics
Heel GmbH
Dr.-Reckeweg-Strasse 2-4
D-76532 Baden-Baden
Germany
Tel: 07221-50100
Fax: 07221-501-208

Pascoe Complex Homeopathics
Pascoe Pharmazeutische
  Präparate GmbH
Schiffenberger Weg 55
D-35394 Giessen
Germany
Tel: 0641-79600
Fax: 0641-796063

EAV Classes
Deutsche Ärztegesellschaft für
  Akupunktur e.V.
Raglovichstrasse 14
80637 München
Germany
Tel: 089-1-59-68-88
Fax: 089-1-59-62-55

Bach Flower Remedies
The Bach Centre
Mount Vernon
Sotwell
Wallingford
OXON OX10 0PZ
UK
Tel: 01491 39489

Protocols for Non-toxic Dentistry
International Academy of Oral
  Medicine and Toxicology
PO Box 608010
Orlando
FL 32860 – 8010
Tel: (407) 290 9670
Fax: (407) 299 4149

Holistic Dental Association
PO Box 5007
Durango, CO 81301
USA

INDEX